T0175675

FIRST AID FOR THE® PSYCHIATRY CLERKSHIP

6th Edition

NOTICE

Medicine is an ever-changing science. As new research and clinical experience broaden our knowledge, changes in treatment and pharmacotherapy are required. The authors and the publisher of this work have checked with sources believed to be reliable in their efforts to provide information that is complete and generally in accord with the standards accepted at the time of publication. However, in view of the possibility of human error or changes in medical sciences, neither the authors nor the publisher nor any other party who has been involved in the preparation or publication of this work warrants that the information contained herein is in every respect accurate or complete, and they disclaim all responsibility for any errors or omissions or for the results obtained from use of the information contained in this work. Readers are encouraged to confirm the information contained herein with other sources. For example and in particular, readers are advised to check the product information sheet included in the package of each medication they plan to administer to be certain that the information contained in this work is accurate and that changes have not been made in the recommended dose or in the contraindications for administration. This recommendation is of particular importance in connection with new or infrequently used drugs.

FIRST AID FOR THE® PSYCHIATRY CLERKSHIP

6th Edition

Sean M. Blitzstein, MD
Staff Psychiatrist
Jesse Brown VA Medical Center
Director, Psychiatry Clerkship
Clinical Professor of Psychiatry
University of Illinois at Chicago
Chicago, Illinois

Latha Ganti, MD, MS, MBA, FACEP, FAHA
Vice Chair for Research and Academic Affairs
HCA UCF Emergency Medicine Residency Program of Greater Orlando
Associate Medical Director, Polk County Fire Rescue
Professor of Emergency Medicine and Neurology
University of Central Florida College of Medicine
Orlando, Florida

Matthew S. Kaufman, MD
Medical Director
Emergency Department
Jersey City Medical Center
Bayonne, New Jersey

New York   Chicago   San Francisco   Athens   London   Madrid   Mexico   City   Milan
New Delhi   Singapore   Sydney   Toronto

First Aid for the® Psychiatry Clerkship, Sixth Edition

Copyright © 2022 by McGraw Hill. All rights reserved. Printed in China. Except as permitted under the United States Copyright Act of 1976, no part of this publication may be reproduced or distributed in any form or by any means, or stored in a data base or retrieval system, without the prior written permission of the publisher.

Previous editions copyright © 2019, 2016 by McGraw-Hill Education and copyright © 2011, 2005, 2002 by The McGraw-Hill Companies, Inc.

First Aid for the® is a registered trademark of McGraw Hill. All rights reserved.

1 2 3 4 5 6 7 8 9 DSS 26 25 24 23 22 21

ISBN 978-1-264-25784-3
MHID 1-264-25784-8

This book was set in Minion Pro by MPS Limited.
The editors were Bob Boehringer and Kim J. Davis.
The production supervisor was Catherine Saggese.
Project management was provided by Adwiti Pradhan.

This book is printed on acid-free paper.

Library of Congress Cataloging-in-Publication Data

Names: Sean M. Blitzstein, author. | Ganti, Latha, author. |
  Kaufman, Matthew S., author.
Title: First aid for the psychiatry clerkship / Latha Ganti, Matthew S.
  Kaufman, Sean M. Blitzstein.
Description: Sixth edition. | New York : McGraw Hill, [2021] | Includes
  index. | Summary: "Each of the chapters in this book contains the major
  topics central to the practice of psychiatry and has been specifically
  designed for the medical student learning level, to excel in the
  clerkship (shelf exams), as well as the USMLE Step 2 and 3 exams"--
  Provided by publisher.
Identifiers: LCCN 2021004054 (print) | LCCN 2021004055 (ebook) | ISBN
  9781264257843 (paperback ; alk. paper) | ISBN 1264257848 (paperback ;
  alk. paper) | ISBN 9781264257850 (ebook) | ISBN 1264257856 (ebook)
Subjects: MESH: Mental Disorders | Clinical Clerkship | Psychiatry |
  Outline
Classification: LCC RC454 (print) | LCC RC454 (ebook) | NLM WM 18.2 |
  DDC 616.89--dc23
LC record available at https://lccn.loc.gov/2021004054
LC ebook record available at https://lccn.loc.gov/2021004055

McGraw Hill books are available at special quantity discounts to use as premiums and sales promotions, or for use in corporate training programs. To contact a representative, please visit the Contact Us pages at www.mhprofessional.com.

CONTENTS

CONTRIBUTING AUTHORS

SEAN M. BLITZSTEIN, MD
Staff Psychiatrist
Jesse Brown VA Medical Center
Director, Psychiatry Clerkship
Clinical Professor of Psychiatry
University of Illinois at Chicago
Chicago, Illinois
Chapter 1: How to Succeed in the Psychiatry Clerkship
Chapter 6: Personality Disorders
Chapter 16: Sexual Dysfunctions and Paraphilic Disorders

LATHA GANTI, MD, MS, MBA, FACEP, FAHA
Vice Chair for Research and Academic Affairs
HCA UCF Emergency Medicine Residency Program of Greater
*   Orlando*
Associate Medical Director, Polk County Fire Rescue
Professor of Emergency Medicine and Neurology
University of Central Florida College of Medicine
Orlando, Florida
Chapter 20: Approach to the Psychiatric Patient in the
*   Emergency Department*

VICTORIA GOTAY, MD
Psychiatry Resident
University of Illinois at Chicago
Chicago, Illinois
Chapter 2: Examination and Diagnosis
Chapter 15: Sleep-Wake Disorders
Chapter 17: Psychotherapies
Chapter 19: Forensic Psychiatry

JACQUELINE HIRSCH, MD
Psychiatry Resident
Department of Psychiatry and Behavioral Sciences
Northwestern University Feinberg School of Medicine
Chicago, Illinois
Chapter 4: Mood Disorders
Chapter 9: Geriatric Psychiatry
Chapter 14: Eating Disorders
Chapter 18: Psychopharmacology

AMBER C. MAY, MD
Child, Adolescent, and Adult Psychiatrist
The Bloomberg Institute
Volunteer Faculty of Clinical Psychiatry & Former Director
*   of the Comprehensive ADHD Clinic*
The University of Illinois at Chicago
Chicago, Illinois
Chapter 5: Anxiety, Obsessive-Compulsive, Trauma, and
*   Stressor-Related Disorders*
Chapter 8: Neurocognitive Disorders
Chapter 10: Psychiatric Disorders in Children
Chapter 11: Dissociative Disorders

SURYA SABHAPATHY, MD, MPH
Assistant Professor of Clinical Psychiatry
Director, Gender and Sexuality Clinic in Psychiatry
University of Illinois at Chicago
Chicago, Illinois
Chapter 3: Psychotic Disorders
Chapter 7: Substance-Related and Addictive Disorders
Chapter 12: Somatic Symptom and Factitious Disorders
Chapter 13: Impulse Control Disorders

CONTRIBUTING AUTHORS

INTRODUCTION

This clinical study aid was designed in the tradition of the First Aid series of books. It is formatted in the same way as the other books in this series. However, a stronger clinical emphasis was placed on its content in relation to psychiatry. You will find that rather than simply preparing you for success on the clerkship exam, this resource will guide you in the clinical diagnosis and treatment of many problems seen by psychiatrists.

Each chapter in this book contains the major topics central to the practice of psychiatry and has been specifically designed for the medical student learning level, to excel in the clerkship (shelf exams), as well as the USMLE Step 2 and 3 exams.

The content of the text is organized in the format similar to other texts in the First Aid series. Topics are listed by bold headings, and the "meat" of the topics provides essential information. The outside margins contain mnemonics, diagrams, exam and ward tips, summary or warning statements, and other memory aids. Exam tips are marked by the ♟ icon, tips for the wards and questions for the wards by the ✋ icon, and clinical scenarios by the ♀ icon.

HOW TO SUCCEED IN THE
PSYCHIATRY CLERKSHIP

Your psychiatry clerkship will undoubtedly be very interesting and exciting. A key to doing well in this clerkship is finding the balance between drawing a firm boundary of professionalism with your patients while maintaining a relationship of trust and empathy.

Why Spend Time on Psychiatry?

For most, your medical school psychiatry clerkship will encompass the entirety of your formal training in psychiatry during your career in medicine.

Being aware of and understanding the features of mental dysfunction in psychiatric patients will serve you well in recognizing psychiatric symptoms in your patients, regardless of your specialty choice.

While anxiety and depression can worsen the prognosis of patients' other medical conditions, medical illnesses can cause significant psychological stress, often uncovering a previously subclinical psychiatric condition. The stress of extended hospitalizations can strain normal mental and emotional functioning beyond their adaptive reserve, resulting in transient psychiatric symptoms.

Psychotropic medications are frequently prescribed in the general population. Many of these drugs have significant medical side effects and drug interactions. You will become familiar with these during your clerkship and will encounter them in clinical practice regardless of your field of medicine.

Because of the unique opportunity to spend a great deal of time interacting with your patients, the psychiatry clerkship is an excellent time to practice your interview skills and "bedside manner."

How to Behave on the Wards

RESPECT THE PATIENTS

Always maintain professionalism and give respect to the patients. Be respectful when discussing cases with your residents and attendings.

RESPECT THE FIELD OF PSYCHIATRY

- Regardless of your interest in psychiatry, take the rotation seriously.
- You may not agree with all the decisions that your residents and attendings make, but it is important for everyone to be on the same page.
- Dress in a professional manner.
- Because of the intense emotional suffering experienced by psychiatric patients, working with them can be overwhelming. Keep yourself healthy.
- Psychiatry is a multidisciplinary field. It would behoove you to continuously communicate with nurses, social workers, and psychologists.
- Address patients formally unless otherwise told.

TAKE RESPONSIBILITY FOR YOUR PATIENTS

Know as much as possible about your patients: their history, psychiatric and medical problems, test results, treatment plan, and prognosis. Keep your intern or resident informed of new developments that they might not be aware of, and ask them for any updates you might not be aware of. Assist the team in developing a plan; speak to consultants and family members. Never deliver bad news to patients or family members without the assistance of your supervising resident or attending.

RESPECT PATIENTS' RIGHTS

1. All patients have the right to have their personal medical information kept private. This means do not discuss the patient's information with family members without that patient's consent, and do not discuss any patient in public areas (e.g., hallways, elevators, cafeterias).
2. All patients have the right to refuse treatment. This means they can refuse treatment by a specific individual (the medical student) or of a specific type (electroconvulsive therapy). Patients can even refuse lifesaving treatment. The only exceptions to this rule are if the patient is deemed to not have the capacity to make decisions or if the patient is suicidal or homicidal.
3. All patients should be informed of the right to seek advance directives on admission. Often, this is done by the admissions staff or by a social worker. If your patient is chronically ill or has a life-threatening illness, address the subject of advance directives with the assistance of your resident or attending.

VOLUNTEER

Be enthusiastic and self-motivated. Volunteer to help with a procedure or a difficult task. Volunteer to give a 20-minute talk on a topic of your choice, to take additional patients, and to stay late.

BE A TEAM PLAYER

Help other medical students with their tasks; teach them information you have learned. Support your supervising intern or resident whenever possible. Never steal the spotlight or make a fellow medical student look bad. If your work for the day is completed, offer to help with tasks on other patients on your team, even if they are not your primary patients; helping to get work done may free up time for the resident or attending to spend more time teaching.

KEEP PATIENT INFORMATION HANDY

Use a clipboard, notebook, or index cards to keep patient information, including a history and physical, lab, and test results, at hand. However, make sure to keep all confidential patient information secure.

PRESENT PATIENT INFORMATION IN AN ORGANIZED MANNER

Here is a template for the "bullet" presentation:

"This is a [**age**]-year-old [**gender**] with a history of [**major history such as bipolar disorder**] who presented on [**date**] with [**major symptoms, such as auditory hallucinations**] and was found to have [**working diagnosis**]. [**Tests done**] showed [**results**]. Yesterday, the patient [**state important changes, new plan, new tests, new medications**]. This morning the patient feels [**state the patient's words**], and the mental status and physical exams are significant for [**state major findings**]. Plan is [**state plan**]."

The newly admitted patient generally deserves a longer presentation following the complete history and physical format.

Many patients have extensive histories. The complete history should be present in the admission note, but during ward presentations, the entire history is often too much to absorb. In these cases, it will be very important that you generate a **good summary** that is concise but maintains an accurate picture of the patient.

How to Prepare for the Clerkship (Shelf) Exam

If you have studied the core psychiatric symptoms and illnesses, you will know a great deal about psychiatry. To specifically study for the clerkship or shelf exam, we recommend:

2–3 weeks before exam: Read this entire review book, taking notes.
10 days before exam: Read the notes you took during the rotation and the corresponding review book sections.
5 days before exam: Read this entire review book, concentrating on lists and mnemonics.
2 days before exam: Exercise, eat well, skim the book, and go to bed early.
1 day before exam: Exercise, eat well, review your notes and the mnemonics, and go to bed on time. Do not have any caffeine after 2 PM.

Other helpful studying strategies are discussed below.

STUDY WITH FRIENDS

Group studying can be very helpful. Other people may point out areas that you have not studied enough and may help you focus more effectively. If you tend to get distracted by other people in the room, limit this amount to less than half of your study time.

STUDY IN A BRIGHT ROOM

Find the room in your home or library that has the brightest light. This will help prevent you from falling asleep. If you don't have a bright light, obtain a halogen desk lamp or a light that simulates sunlight.

EAT LIGHT, BALANCED MEALS

Make sure your meals are balanced, with lean protein, fruits and vegetables, and fiber. A high-sugar, high-carbohydrate meal will give you an initial burst of energy for 1–2 hours, but then your blood sugar will quickly drop.

UTILIZE QUESTION BANKS AND/OR TAKE PRACTICE EXAMS

The purpose of practice exams is not just for the content that is contained in the questions, but the process of sitting for several hours and attempting to choose the best answer for each and every question.

POCKET CARDS

The "cards" on the following page contain information that is often helpful in psychiatry practice. We advise that you make a photocopy of these cards, cut them out, and carry them with you.

Mental Status Exam

Appearance/Behavior: Apparent age, attitude and cooperativeness, eye contact, posture, dress and hygiene, psychomotor status.

Speech: Rate, rhythm, volume, tone, articulation.

Mood: Patient's subjective emotional state—depressed, anxious, sad, angry, etc.

Affect: Objective emotional expression—euthymic, dysphoric, euphoric, appropriate (to stated mood), labile, full, constricted, flat, etc.

Thought process: Logical/linear, circumstantial, tangential, flight of ideas, looseness of association, thought blocking.

Thought content: Suicidal/homicidal ideation, delusions, ideas of reference, paranoia, obsessions, preoccupations, hyperreligiosity.

Perceptual disturbances: Hallucinations, illusions, derealization, depersonalization.

Cognition:

Level of consciousness: Alert, sleepy, lethargic.

Orientation: Person, place, date.

Attention/Concentration: Serial 7s, spell "world" backward.

Abstract thought: Interpretation of proverbs, analogies.

Memory:

Registration: Immediate recall of three objects.

Short term: Recall of objects after 5 minutes.

Long term: Ask about verifiable personal information.

Fund of knowledge: Current events.

Insight: Patient's awareness of their illness and need for treatment.

Judgment: Patient's ability to approach their problems in an appropriate manner.

Delirium

Characteristics: Acute onset, waxing/waning sensorium (worse at night), disorientation, inattention, impaired cognition, disorganized thinking, altered sleep-wake cycle, perceptual disorders (hallucinations, illusions).

Etiology: Drugs (narcotics, benzodiazepines, anticholinergics [e.g., diphenhydramine], TCAs, steroids), EtOH withdrawal, metabolic (cardiac, respiratory, renal, hepatic, endocrine), infection, neurological causes (increased ICP, encephalitis, postictal, stroke).

Investigations:

Routine: CBC, chemistry panel, glucose, LFTs, TFTs, thiamine, folate, UA, urine toxicology screen, CXR, vital signs.

Medium-yield: ABG, ECG (silent MI), ionized Ca^{2+}.

If above inconclusive: Head CT/MRI, EEG, LP.

Management: Identify/correct underlying cause, simplify Rx regimen, discontinue potentially offensive medications if possible, avoid benzodiazepines (except in EtOH withdrawal), create safe environment, provide reassurance/education, judiciously use antipsychotics for acute agitation.

Mini-Mental State Examination (MMSE)

Orientation (10):

What is the [year] [season] [date] [day] [month]? (1 pt. each)

Where are we [state] [county] [town] [hospital] [floor]?

Registration (3): Ask the patient to repeat three unrelated objects (1 pt. each on first attempt). If incomplete on first attempt, repeat up to six times (record number of trials).

Attention (5): Either serial 7s or spell "world" backward (1 pt. for each correct letter or number).

Delayed recall (3): Ask patient to recall the three objects previously named (1 pt. each).

Language (9):

- Name two common objects, e.g., watch, pen (1 pt. each).
- Repeat the following sentence: "No ifs, ands, or buts" (1 pt.).
- Give patient blank paper. "Take it in your right hand, use both hands to fold it in half, and then put it on the floor" (1 pt. for each part correctly executed).
- Have patient read and follow: "Close your eyes" (1 pt.).
- Ask patient to write a sentence. The sentence must contain a subject and a verb; correct grammar and punctuation are not necessary (1 pt.).
- Ask the patient to copy the design. Each figure must have five sides, and two of the angles must intersect (1 pt.).

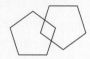

Mania ("DIG FAST")

Distractibility

Irritable mood/insomnia

Grandiosity

Flight of ideas

Agitation/increase in goal-directed activity

Speedy thoughts/speech

Thoughtlessness: seek pleasure without regard to consequences

Suicide Risk ("SAD PERSONS")

Sex—Male

Age >60 years

Depression

Previous attempt

Ethanol/drug abuse

Rational thinking loss

Suicide in family

Organized plan/access

No support

Sickness

Major Depression ("SIG E. CAPS")

Sleep

Interest

Guilt

Energy

Concentration

Appetite

Psychomotor Δs

Suicidal ideation

- Hopelessness
- Helplessness
- Worthlessness

Drugs of Abuse		
Drug	**Intoxication**	**Withdrawal**
Alcohol benzodiazepines	Disinhibition, mood lability, incoordination, slurred speech, ataxia, blackouts (EtOH), respiratory depression	Tremulousness, hypertension, tachycardia, anxiety, psychomotor agitation, nausea, seizures, hallucinations, DTs (EtOH)
Barbiturates	Respiratory depression	Anxiety, seizures, delirium, life-threatening cardiovascular collapse
Opioids	CNS depression, nausea, vomiting, sedation, decreased pain perception, decreased GI motility, pupil constriction, respiratory depression	Increased sympathetic activity, N/V, diarrhea, diaphoresis, rhinorrhea, piloerection, yawning, stomach cramps, myalgias, arthralgias, restlessness, anxiety, anorexia
Amphetamines cocaine	Euphoria, increased attention span, aggressiveness, psychomotor agitation, pupil dilatation, hypertension, tachycardia, cardiac arrhythmias, psychosis, formication with cocaine	Post-use "crash": restlessness, headache, hunger, severe depression, irritability, insomnia/hypersomnia, strong psychological craving
PCP	Belligerence, impulsiveness, psychomotor agitation, vertical/horizontal nystagmus, hyperthermia, tachycardia, ataxia, psychosis, homicidality	May have recurrence of symptoms due to reabsorption in GI tract
LSD	Altered perceptual states (hallucinations, distortions of time and space), elevation of mood, "bad trips" (panic reaction), flashbacks (reexperience of the sensations in absence of drug use)	
Cannabis	Euphoria, anxiety, paranoia, slowed time, social withdrawal, increased appetite, dry mouth, tachycardia, amotivational syndrome	
Nicotine/Caffeine	Restlessness, insomnia, anxiety, anorexia	Irritability, lethargy, headache, increased appetite, weight gain

First Aid for the Psychiatry Clerkship, 4e; copyright © 2015 McGraw-Hill. All rights reserved.

Psychiatric Emergencies

Delirium Tremens (DTs):

- Typically within 2–4 days after cessation of EtOH but may occur later.
- Delirium, agitation, fever, autonomic hyperactivity, auditory and visual hallucinations.
- Treat aggressively with benzodiazepines and hydration.

Neuroleptic Malignant Syndrome (NMS):

- Fever, rigidity, autonomic instability, clouding of consciousness, elevated WBC/CPK.
- Withhold neuroleptics, hydrate, consider dantrolene, and/or bromocriptine.
- Idiosyncratic, time-limited reaction.

Serotonin Syndrome:

- Precipitated by use of two drugs with serotonin-enhancing properties (e.g., MAOI + SSRI).
- Altered mental status, fever, agitation, tremor, myoclonus, hyperreflexia, ataxia, incoordination, diaphoresis, shivering, diarrhea.
- Discontinue offending agents, benzodiazepines, consider cyproheptadine.

Tyramine Reaction/Hypertensive Crisis:

- Precipitated by ingestion of tyramine-containing foods while on MAOIs.
- Hypertension, headache, neck stiffness, sweating, nausea, vomiting, visual problems. Most serious consequences are stroke and possibly death.
- Treat with nitroprusside or phentolamine.

Acute Dystonia:

- Early, sudden onset of muscle spasm: eyes, tongue, jaw, neck; may lead to laryngospasm requiring intubation.
- Treat with benztropine (Cogentin) or diphenhydramine (Benadryl).
- If clinically appropriate, reduce the dose, discontinue the medication, or switch to another agent.

Lithium Toxicity:

- May occur at any Li level (usually >1.5).
- Nausea, vomiting, slurred speech, ataxia, incoordination, myoclonus, hyperreflexia, seizures, nephrogenic diabetes insipidus, delirium, coma.
- Discontinue Li, hydrate aggressively, consider hemodialysis.

Tricyclic Antidepressant (TCA) Toxicity:

- Primarily anticholinergic effects, cardiac conduction disturbances, hypotension, respiratory depression, agitation, hallucinations, seizures.
- Classic ECG finding is QRS >100 ms.
- Treatment includes sodium bicarbonate, activated charcoal, cathartics, supportive treatment.
- Discontinue the medication.

CHAPTER 2

EXAMINATION AND
DIAGNOSIS

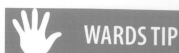

WARDS TIP

The history of present illness (HPI) should include information about the current episode, including symptoms, duration, context, stressors, and impairment in function.

WARDS TIP

If you are seeing the patient in the ER, make sure to ask how they got to the ER (police, bus, walk-in, family member) and look to see what time they were triaged. For all initial evaluations, ask why the patient is seeking treatment **today** as opposed to any other day.

WARDS TIP

When taking a substance history, remember to ask about caffeine and nicotine use. If a heavy smoker is hospitalized and does not have access to nicotine replacement therapy, nicotine withdrawal may cause anxiety and agitation.

History and Mental Status Examination

INTERVIEWING

Making the Patient Comfortable

The initial interview is of utmost importance to the psychiatrist. With practice, you will develop your own style and learn how to adapt the interview to the individual patient. In general, start the interview by asking open-ended questions. Carefully note how the patient responds, as this is critical information for the mental status exam. Consider preparing for the interview by writing down the subheadings of the exam (see Figure 2-1). Find a safe and private area to conduct the interview. Use closed-ended questions to obtain the remaining pertinent information. During the first interview, the psychiatrist must establish a meaningful rapport with the patient in order to get accurate and pertinent information. This requires that the questions be asked in a quiet, comfortable setting so that the patient is at ease. The patient should feel that the psychiatrist is interested, nonjudgmental, and compassionate. In psychiatry, the history is the most important factor in formulating a diagnosis and treatment plan.

Date and Location:

Identifying Patient Data:

Chief Complaint: Past Medical History:

History of Present Illness:

                                                   Allergies:

Past Psychiatric History: Current Meds:

First contact:

Diagnosis: Developmental History:

Prior hospitalizations:

Suicide attempts: Relationships (children/marital status):

Outpatient treatment:

Med trials: Education:

                                                   Work History:

Substance History: Military History:

                                                   Housing:

Smoking: Income:

Family Psychiatric History: Religion:

Legal History:

FIGURE 2-1. Psychiatric history outline.

TAKING THE HISTORY

The psychiatric history follows a similar format as the history for other types of patients. It should include the following:

- Identifying data: The patient's name, preferred gender, age, marital status.

- Chief complaint (use the patient's own words): If called as a consultant, list reason for the consult.

- Sources of information.

- History of present illness (HPI):

  - *The 4 Ps:* The patient's psychosocial and environmental conditions *predisposing to, precipitating, perpetuating,* and *protecting* against the current episode.

  - The patient's support system (whom the patient lives with, distance and level of contact with friends and relatives).

  - Neurovegetative symptoms (quality of sleep, appetite, energy, psychomotor retardation/activation, concentration).

  - Suicidal ideation/homicidal ideation.

  - How work and relationship have been affected (for most diagnoses in the *Diagnostic and Statistical Manual of Mental Disorders,* 5th edition [*DSM-5*] there is a criterion that specifies that symptoms must cause clinically significant distress or impairment in social, occupational, or other important areas of functioning).

  - Psychotic symptoms (e.g., auditory and visual hallucinations, delusions).

  - Establish a baseline of mental health:

    - Patient's level of functioning when "well."

    - Goals (outpatient setting).

- Past psychiatric history (include as applicable: history of suicide attempts, history of self-harm [e.g., cutting, burning oneself], information about previous episodes, other psychiatric disorders in remission, medication trials, past psychiatric hospitalizations, current outpatient psychiatrist).

- Substance history (age of first use, amount and route of use, history of withdrawal/delirium tremens (DTs), longest period of sobriety, history of intravenous drug use, participation in outpatient or inpatient drug rehab programs).

- Medical history (ask specifically about head trauma, seizures, pregnancy status).

- Family psychiatric and medical history (include substance use, suicides, and response to specific psychotropic agents as patient may respond similarly).

- Medications (ask about supplements and over-the-counter [OTC] medications, as well as compliance).

- Allergies: Clarify if it was a true allergy or an adverse drug event (e.g., abdominal pain).

- Developmental/Social history: Achieved developmental milestones on time, friends in school, history of trauma or abuse, performance academically. Also include income source, employment, education, place of residence, who they live with, number of children, support system, religious affiliation and beliefs, legal history, and amount of exercise.

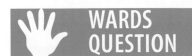

WARDS QUESTION

Q: What OTC medication would be important to ask and document in a patient with bipolar disorder taking Lithium.
A: Nonsteroidal anti-inflammatory drugs (NSAIDs) as they can ↑ lithium concentrations.

WARDS TIP

Psychomotor retardation, which refers to the slowness of voluntary and involuntary movements, may also be referred to as hypokinesia or bradykinesia. The term akinesia is used in extreme cases where absence of movement is observed.

KEY FACT

Automatisms are spontaneous, involuntary movements that occur during an altered state of consciousness and can range from purposeful to disorganized.

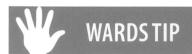

WARDS QUESTION

Q: What is pressured speech?
A: Speech that is usually uninterruptible with the patient compelled to continue speaking.

WARDS TIP

To assess mood, ask, "How are you feeling today?" It can also be helpful to have patients rate their stated mood on a scale of 1–10.

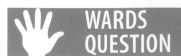

WARDS QUESTION

Q: What is a flat affect?
A: A patient who remains expressionless and monotone even when discussing extremely sad or happy moments in their life.

MENTAL STATUS EXAMINATION

This is analogous to performing a physical exam in other areas of medicine. It is the nuts and bolts of the psychiatric exam. It should describe the patient in as much detail as possible. The mental status exam assesses the following:

- Appearance/Behavior
- Speech
- Mood/Affect
- Thought process
- Thought content
- Perceptual disturbances
- Cognition
- Insight
- Judgment/Impulse control

The mental status exam tells only about the mental status at that moment; it can change every hour or every day, etc.

Appearance/Behavior

- *Appearance:* Gender, age (looks older/younger than stated age), type of clothing, hygiene (including smelling of alcohol, urine, feces), posture, grooming, physical abnormalities, tattoos, body piercings. Take specific notice of the following, which may be clues for possible diagnoses:
  - Pupil size: Drug intoxication/withdrawal.
  - Bruises in hidden areas: ↑ suspicion for abuse.
  - Needle marks/tracks: Drug use.
  - Eroding of tooth enamel: Eating disorders (from vomiting).
  - Superficial cuts on arms: Self-harm.
- *Behavior:* Attitude (cooperative, seductive, flattering, charming, eager to please, entitled, controlling, uncooperative, hostile, guarded, critical, antagonistic, childish), positioning (sitting, standing), mannerisms, tics, eye contact, activity level, psychomotor retardation/activation, akathisia, automatisms, catatonia, choreoathetoid movements, compulsions, dystonias, tremor.

Speech

Rate (pressured, slowed, regular), rhythm (i.e., prosody), articulation (dysarthria, stuttering), accent/dialect, volume/modulation (loudness or softness), tone, long or short latency of speech, quantity of speech (hyperverbal, paucity of speech).

Mood

Mood is the emotion that the patient tells you they feel, often in quotations.

Affect

Affect is an assessment of how the patient's mood appears to the examiner, including the amount and range of emotional expression. It is described with the following dimensions:

- *Type of affect:* Euthymic, euphoric, neutral, dysphoric.
- *Range* describes the depth and range of the feelings shown. Parameters: flat (none)—blunted (shallow)—constricted (limited)—full (average)—intense (more than normal).
- *Motility* describes how quickly a person appears to shift emotional states. Parameters: sluggish—supple—labile.

- *Appropriateness to content* describes whether the affect is congruent with the subject of conversation or stated mood. Parameters: appropriate—not appropriate.

Thought Process

The patient's form of thinking—how they use language and put ideas together. It describes whether the patient's thoughts are logical, meaningful, and goal directed. It does not comment on *what* the patient thinks, only *how* the patient expresses their thoughts.

- **Logical/Linear/Goal-directed:** Answers to questions and conversation clear and follows a logical sequence.
- **Circumstantiality** is when the point of the conversation is eventually reached but with overinclusion of trivial or irrelevant details.

Examples of thought disorders include:

- **Tangentiality:** Can follow conversation but point never reached or question never answered.
- **Loosening of associations:** No logical connection from one thought to another.
- **Flight of ideas:** Thoughts change abruptly from one idea to another, often based on understandable associations or distracting stimuli; usually accompanied by rapid/pressured speech.
- **Neologisms:** Made-up words.
- **Word salad:** Incoherent collection of words.
- **Clang associations:** Word connections due to phonetics rather than actual meaning. "My car is red. I've been in bed. It hurts my head."
- **Thought blocking:** Abrupt cessation of communication before the idea is finished.

Thought Content

Describes the types of ideas expressed by the patient. Examples of disorders:

- **Poverty of thought versus overabundance:** Too few versus too many ideas expressed.
- **Delusions:** Fixed, false beliefs that are not shared by the person's culture and remain despite evidence to the contrary. Delusions are classified as bizarre (impossible to be true) or nonbizarre (at least possible).
- **Suicidal and homicidal ideation:** Ask if the patient feels like harming themself or others. Identify if the plan is well formulated. Ask if the patient has an intent (i.e., if released right now, would they kill themself or harm others?). Ask if the patient has means to kill themself (firearms in the house/multiple prescription bottles).
- **Phobias:** Persistent, irrational fears.
- **Obsessions:** Repetitive, intrusive thoughts.

Perceptual Disturbances

- *Hallucinations:* Sensory perceptions that occur in the absence of an actual stimulus.
  - Describe the sensory modality: Auditory (most common), visual, gustatory, olfactory, or tactile.
  - Describe the details (e.g., auditory hallucinations may be ringing, humming, whispers, or voices speaking clear words). Command auditory hallucinations are voices that instruct the patient to do something.

KEY FACT

An example of inappropriate affect is a patient's laughing when being told they have a serious illness.

WARDS TIP

A patient who is laughing one second and crying the next has a *labile* affect.

KEY FACT

Examples of delusions:

- *Grandeur*—Belief that one has special powers or is someone important (Jesus, President).
- *Paranoid*—Belief that one is being persecuted.
- *Reference*—Belief that some event is uniquely related to patient (e.g., a TV show character is sending messages to patient).
- *Thought broadcasting*—Belief that one's thoughts can be heard by others.
- *Religious*—Conventional beliefs exaggerated (e.g., God wants me to be the Messiah).
- *Somatic*—False belief concerning body image (e.g., I have cancer).

WARDS TIP

The following question can help screen for obsessions: Do you think and/or worry about checking, cleaning, or counting on a repetitive basis?

WARDS QUESTION

Q: What type of hallucinations are an important risk factor for suicide or homicide?
A: Command hallucinations (auditory hallucinations that instruct a patient to harm themselves or others).

WARDS TIP

Alcoholic hallucinosis refers to hallucinations (usually auditory, although visual and tactile may occur) that occur either during or after a period of heavy alcohol consumption. Patients usually are aware that these hallucinations are not real. In contrast to DTs, there is no clouding of sensorium and vital signs are normal.

KEY FACT

You can roughly assess a patient's intellectual functioning by utilizing the **proverb interpretation** and **vocabulary** strategies. Proverb interpretation is helpful in assessing whether a patient has difficulty with abstraction. Being able to define a particular vocabulary word correctly and appropriately and use it in a sentence reflects a person's intellectual capacity.

- Ask if the hallucination is experienced only while falling asleep (hypnagogic hallucination) or upon awakening (hypnopompic hallucination).
- *Illusions:* Inaccurate perception of existing sensory stimuli (e.g., wall appears as if it's moving).
- *Derealization/Depersonalization:* The experience of feeling detached from one's surroundings/mental processes.

Cognition

- **Consciousness:** Patient's level of awareness; possible range includes: alert—drowsy—lethargic—stuporous—comatose.
- **Orientation:** To person, place, and time.
- **Calculation:** Ability to add/subtract.
- **Memory:**
  - Immediate (registration)—Dependent on attention/concentration and can be tested by asking a patient to repeat several digits or words.
  - Recent (short-term memory)—Events within the past few minutes, hours, or days.
  - Remote memory (long-term memory).
- **Fund of knowledge:** Level of knowledge in the context of the patient's culture and education (e.g., Who is the president? Who was Picasso?).
- **Attention/Concentration:** Ability to subtract serial 7s from 100 or to spell "world" backward.
- **Reading/Writing:** Simple sentences (must make sure the patient is literate first).
- **Abstract concepts:** Ability to explain similarities between objects and understand the meaning of simple proverbs.

Insight

Insight is the patient's level of awareness and understanding of their problem. Problems with insight include complete denial of illness or blaming it on something else. Insight can be described as full, partial/limited, or minimal.

Judgment

Judgment is the patient's ability to understand the outcome of their actions and use this awareness in decision making; it is best determined from information from the HPI and recent behavior (e.g., how a patient was brought to treatment or medication compliance). Judgment can be described as excellent, good, fair, or poor.

 Mrs. W is a 52-year-old female who arrives at the emergency room reporting that her deceased husband of 25 years told her that he would be waiting for her there. To meet him, she drove nonstop for 22 hours from a nearby state. She claims that her husband is a famous preacher and that she, too, has a mission from God. Although she does not specify the details of her mission, she says that she was given the ability to stop time until her mission is completed. She reports experiencing high levels of energy despite not sleeping for 22 hours. She also reports that she has a history of psychiatric hospitalizations but refuses to provide further information.

While obtaining her history you perform a mental status exam. Her **appearance** is that of a woman who looks older than her stated age. She is obese and unkempt. There is no evidence of tattoos or piercings. She has tousled hair and is dressed in a mismatched flowered skirt and a red T-shirt. Upon her arrival at the emergency room, her **behavior** is demanding, as she insists that you let her husband know that she has arrived. She then becomes irate and proceeds to yell, banging her head against the wall. She screams, "Stop hiding him from me!" She is uncooperative with redirection and is guarded during the remainder of the interview. Her eye contact is poor as she is looking around the room. Her **psychomotor activity** is agitated. Her **speech** is loud and pressured, with a foreign accent.

She reports that her **mood** is "angry," and her **affect** as observed during the interview is labile and irritable.

Her **thought process** includes flight of ideas. Her **thought content** is significant for delusions of grandeur and thought broadcasting, as evidenced by her refusing to answer most questions claiming that you are able to know what she is thinking. She denies suicidal or homicidal ideation. She expresses **disturbances in perception** as she admits to frequent auditory hallucinations without commands.

She is uncooperative with formal **cognitive** testing, but you notice that she is oriented to place and person. However, she erroneously states that it is 2005. Her attention and concentration are notably impaired, as she appears distracted and frequently needs questions repeated. Her **insight, judgment, and impulse control** are determined to be poor.

You decide to admit Mrs. W to the inpatient psychiatric unit in order to allow for comprehensive diagnostic evaluation, the opportunity to obtain collateral information from her prior hospitalizations, safety monitoring, medical workup for possible reversible causes of her symptoms, and psychopharmacological treatment.

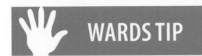

WARDS TIP

To test ability to abstract, ask:

1. Similarities: How are an apple and orange alike? (Normal answer: "They are fruits." **Concrete** answer: "They are round.")
2. Proverb testing: What is meant by the phrase, "You can't judge a book by its cover?" (Normal answer: "You can't judge people just by how they look." **Concrete** answer: "Books have different covers.")

BEDSIDE COGNITIVE TESTING

The Montreal Cognitive Assessment (MoCA)
The MoCA is a simple, brief test used to assess gross cognitive functioning. The test and its instructions are available online (Figure 2-2). The areas tested include:

- Orientation (to person, place, and time).
  - Memory (immediate—repeating five words; and recent—recalling the words 5 minutes later).
  - Attention (serial 7s, tapping hand with certain letters, repeating digits).
  - Language (naming, repetition, fluency).
  - Abstraction (e.g., saying how a "train" and "bicycle" are alike).
  - Visuospatial ability/executive functioning (trail making task, cube copying, clock drawing).

The Mini-Mental State Examination (MMSE)
The MMSE is another test of cognition that can be performed in a few minutes at the bedside. Unlike the MoCA, the MMSE is copyright protected.

KEY FACT

A prior history of violence is the most important predictor of future violence.

MONTREAL COGNITIVE ASSESSMENT (MoCA®)
Version 8.1 English

Name:
Education:
Sex:
Date of birth:
DATE:

VISUOSPATIAL/EXECUTIVE		POINTS

Copy cube

Draw CLOCK (Ten past eleven)
(3 points)

[ ]

[ ]   [ ] Contour   [ ] Numbers   [ ] Hands   __/5

NAMING

[ ]   [ ]   [ ]   __/3

MEMORY	Read list of words, subject must repeat them. Do 2 trials, even if 1st trial is successful. Do a recall after 5 minutes.		FACE	VELVET	CHURCH	DAISY	RED	
		1ST TRIAL						NO POINTS
		2ND TRIAL						

ATTENTION	Read list of digits (1 digit/ sec.).	Subject has to repeat them in the forward order. [ ] 2 1 8 5 4	
		Subject has to repeat them in the backward order. [ ] 7 4 2	__/2

Read list of letters. The subject must tap with his hand at each letter A. No points if ≥ 2 errors
[ ] F B A C M N A A J K L B A F A K D E A A A J A M O F A A B   __/1

Serial 7 subtraction starting at 100. [ ] 93 [ ] 86 [ ] 79 [ ] 72 [ ] 65
4 or 5 correct subtractions: **3 pts,** 2 or 3 correct: **2 pts,** 1 correct: **1 pt,** 0 correct: **0**   __/3

LANGUAGE	Repeat: I only know that John is the one to help today. [ ]	
	The cat always hid under the couch when dogs were in the room. [ ]	__/2

Fluency: Name maximum number of words in one minute that begin with the letter F. [ ] _____ (N ≥ 11 words)   __/1

ABSTRACTION	Similarity between e.g. orange - banana = fruit [ ] train - bicycle [ ] watch - ruler	__/2

DELAYED RECALL	(MIS)	Has to recall words WITH NO CUE	FACE [ ]	VELVET [ ]	CHURCH [ ]	DAISY [ ]	RED [ ]	Points for UNCUED recall only	__/5
Memory Index Score (MIS)	X3								
	X2	Category cue							
	X1	Multiple choice cue					MIS = ____ /15		

ORIENTATION	[ ] Date [ ] Month [ ] Year [ ] Day [ ] Place [ ] City	__/6

© Z. Nasreddine MD
Administered by: _____
Training and Certification are required to ensure accuracy

www.mocatest.org

MIS: /15
(Normal ≥ 26/30)
Add 1 point if ≤ 12 yr edu

TOTAL   __/30

FIGURE 2-2. Montreal Cognitive Assessment Test (MoCA). Copyright © Z. Nasreddine MD. Reproduced with permission. Copies are available at www.mocatest.org.

Sample Write-Up

CHIEF COMPLAINT: "I'm in despair and hopeless"

HISTORY OF PRESENT ILLNESS:
A 58 year-old domiciled, recently unemployed, single female with a past psychiatric history of depression and no past medical history who presented to the emergency room for depression and suicidal ideation with a plan to jump in front of a train.

The patient explained that she was working as an Licensed Practical Nurse (LPN) for a nursing home when the coronavirus pandemic began. She currently lives with her mother and brother. Her mother is elderly with chronic medical conditions, so they serve as her caretakers. When patients and staff at the nursing home began to test positive for COVID, the patient's brother urged her to quit, given her elevated risk of infection and potential spread to the rest of her family.

She therefore quit her job and has been staying at home with her mother in quarantine for 4 months. For the past 2 months, she has noticed a decline in her mood. She describes feeling "in despair and hopeless…I feel so useless now." She has also been experiencing hypersomnia with worsening fatigue, poor appetite, anhedonia, anergia, and difficulty concentrating. She expressed that for the past 2 weeks she has had suicidal ideation with a plan to jump in front of the train near her home. She denies preparatory behaviors or prior suicide attempts. She denies self-harm behaviors. She realized she needed help now because the suicidal thoughts were becoming more persistent. She notes that her family is what has prevented her from acting on these thoughts. She denies any auditory/visual hallucinations, clustered manic symptoms, or homicidal ideation. She denies any illicit drug or alcohol use.

Of note, for the past week, she has been taking a friend's sertraline to help with her mood.

Patient was amenable to inpatient psychiatric admission. She was agreeable to starting sertraline for her depression.

PAST PSYCHIATRIC HISTORY:
Diagnoses: Depression

Prior Hospitalizations: One time at age 38 for similar symptoms of depression. She was treated with sertraline 50 mg with significant improvement in her symptoms. She continued medications and outpatient therapy for 1 year, but she discontinued both because her depressive symptoms resolved.

Prior Self-Injury: No history of suicide attempts or self-harm

SUBSTANCE USE:
- Tobacco: Smokes 1/2 pack per day
- Alcohol: None
- Illicits: None
- Rehabilitation: Denies

PAST MEDICAL HISTORY:
None. No history of seizures or head trauma.

MEDICATIONS: Sertraline 50 mg daily

ALLERGIES: No known drug allergies

FAMILY HISTORY: Mother with depression but not treated. No history of suicide attempts.

SOCIAL HISTORY
- Lives with brother and mother in apartment
- No history of physical or sexual abuse.
- Development: Met all milestones on time
- Employment: Was working as LPN at a nursing home, currently unemployed
- Education: 2 years of college
- Relationship: Single, never married, no children
- Legal: No legal problems

MENTAL STATUS EXAM
- Appearance: Medium-built female, dressed in hospital gown, good grooming and hygiene, appears consistent with stated age
- Behavior: Sitting comfortably, cooperative during interview, attentive, maintains appropriate eye contact; some psychomotor retardation, no abnormal movements/tics
- Speech: Increased speech latency, low tone, normal prosody
- Mood: "Hopeless"
- Affect: Dysphoric, constricted, congruent with stated mood, non-labile
- Thought Process: Linear, logical, goal-directed
- Thought Content: +Suicidal ideation with plan to jump in front of train, denies homicidal ideation, paranoia, or delusions
- Perceptions: Denies auditory or visual hallucinations and does not appear to be responding to abnormal internal stimuli
- Cognition: Alert and oriented to person, place, and time; memory intact to recent/remote events, good attention (able to do serial 7s)
- Insight: Good—realizes she is having similar symptoms to prior episode of depression related to job loss and isolation.
- Judgement: Fair—brought herself in when she was feeling more suicidal but taking friend's sertraline.

ASSESSMENT:
Patient is a 58 year-old, domiciled, recently unemployed, single female with a past psychiatric history of depression and no past medical history who presented to the emergency room for depression and suicidal ideation with a plan to jump in front of a train. Biologically, she has a first-degree parent (mother) with a history of depression. She denies illicit drug use or alcohol use, therefore not a substance-induced mood disorder. She has a history of depression, and currently has major neurovegetative signs and symptoms consistent with another major depressive episode. She has suicidal ideation with a plan to jump in front of a train and is therefore at high acute risk of harm to self. Psychosocially, her recent unemployment and home quarantine due to the coronavirus was the catalyst for her current mood disturbance. She requires inpatient hospitalization for acute safety/stabilization as she poses a significant risk of harm to herself.

Principal *DSM-5* diagnosis:
Major depressive disorder, recurrent, severe
PLAN:
- Admit to inpatient psychiatry
- Vitals: Per ward routine
- Labs: Chemistry panel, complete blood count, urine toxicology screen, blood alcohol level, thyroid panel
- Diet: General
- Activity: Up ad lib

Depression
- Start sertraline 50 mg daily given prior benefit and tolerability

Tobacco Use
- Offer nicotine replacement (e.g., nicotine patch/gum)

#Social/disposition: Consider family meeting, refer to outpatient medication management, consider psychotherapy

Interviewing Skills

GENERAL APPROACHES TO TYPES OF PATIENTS

Violent Patient

Do not interview a potentially violent patient alone. Inform staff of your whereabouts. Know if there are accessible panic buttons. To assess violence or homicidality, one can simply ask, "Do you feel like you want to hurt someone or that you might hurt someone?" If the patient expresses imminent threats against specific friends, family, or others, the doctor must notify potential victims and/or protection agencies (Tarasoff Rule).

Delusional Patient

Although you should not directly challenge a delusion or insist that it is untrue, you should not imply you believe it either; you should simply acknowledge that you understand that the *patient believes* the delusion is true.

Depressed Patient

A depressed patient may be skeptical that they can be helped. It is important to offer reassurance that they can improve with appropriate therapy. Inquiring about suicidal thoughts is crucial; a feeling of hopelessness, substance use, and/or a history of prior suicide attempts reveal an ↑ risk for suicide. If the patient is actively planning or contemplating suicide, they should be hospitalized or otherwise protected.

Diagnosis and Classification

DIAGNOSIS AS PER *DSM-5*

The American Psychiatric Association (APA) uses a criterion-based system for diagnoses. Criteria and codes for each diagnosis are outlined in the *DSM-5*.

Diagnostic Testing

INTELLIGENCE TESTS

Aspects of intelligence include memory, logical reasoning, ability to assimilate factual knowledge, and understanding of abstract concepts.

Intelligence Quotient (IQ)

IQ is a test of intelligence with a mean of 100 and a standard deviation of 15. These scores are adjusted for age. An IQ of 100 signifies that mental age equals chronological age and corresponds to the 50th percentile in intellectual ability for the general population.

Intelligence tests assess cognitive function by evaluating comprehension, fund of knowledge, math skills, vocabulary, picture assembly, and other verbal and performance skills. Two common tests are:

Wechsler Adult Intelligence Scale (WAIS):

- Most common test for ages 16–90.
- Assesses overall intellectual functioning.
- Four index scores: Verbal comprehension, perceptual reasoning, working memory, processing speed.

Wechsler Intelligence Scale for Children (WISC): Tests intellectual ability in patients ages 6–16.

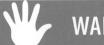

WARDS TIP

In assessing suicidality, do not simply ask, "Do you want to hurt yourself?" because this does not directly address suicidality (they may plan on dying in a painless way). Ask directly about killing self or suicide. If contemplating suicide, ask the patient if they have a plan of how to do it and if they have intent; a detailed plan, intent, and the means to accomplish it suggest a serious threat.

KEY FACT

The Minnesota Multiphasic Personality Inventory (MMPI) is an objective psychological test that is used to assess a person's personality and identify psychopathologies. The mean score for each scale is 50 and the standard deviation is 10.

WARDS TIP

IQ Chart
Very superior: >130
Superior: 120–129
High average: 110–119
Average: 90–109
Low average: 80–89
Borderline: 70–79
Extremely low (intellectual disability): <70

OBJECTIVE PERSONALITY ASSESSMENT TESTS

These tests are questions with standardized-answer format that are objectively scored. The following is an example:

Minnesota Multiphasic Personality Inventory (MMPI-2)
- Tests personality for different pathologies and behavioral patterns.
- Most commonly used.

PROJECTIVE (PERSONALITY) ASSESSMENT TESTS

Projective tests have no structured-response format. The tests often ask for interpretation of ambiguous stimuli. Examples are:

Thematic Apperception Test (TAT)
- Test taker creates stories based on pictures of people in various situations.
- Used to evaluate motivations behind behaviors.

Rorschach Test
- Interpretation of inkblots.
- Used to identify thought disorders and defense mechanisms.

CHAPTER 3

PSYCHOTIC DISORDERS

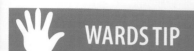

WARDS TIP

Psychosis is exemplified by delusions, hallucinations, or severe disorganization of thought/behavior.

Psychosis

Psychosis is a general term used to describe a distorted perception of reality. Poor reality testing may be accompanied by delusions, perceptual disturbances (illusions or hallucinations), and/or disorganized thinking/behavior. Psychosis can be a symptom of schizophrenia, mania, depression, delirium, and major neurocognitive disorder (i.e., dementia), and it can be substance or medication-induced.

DELUSIONS

Delusions are fixed, false beliefs that persist despite evidence to the contrary and that do not make sense within the context of an individual's cultural background.

They can be categorized as either bizarre or nonbizarre. A *nonbizarre* delusion is a false belief that is plausible but is not true. Example: "The neighbors are spying on me by reading my e-mail." A *bizarre* delusion is a false belief that is impossible. Example: "Aliens are spying on me through a Wi-Fi connection in my brain."

Delusions can also be categorized by theme:

- **Delusions of persecution/paranoid delusions:** Irrational belief that one is being persecuted. Example: "The Central Intelligence Agency (CIA) is monitoring me and tapped my cell phone."
- **Delusions of reference:** Belief that cues in the external environment are uniquely related to the individual. Example: "The TV characters are speaking directly to me."
- **Delusions of control:** Includes **thought broadcasting** (belief that one's thoughts can be heard by others) and **thought insertion** (belief that outside thoughts are being placed in one's head).
- **Delusions of grandeur:** Belief that one has special powers beyond those of a normal person. Example: "I am the all-powerful son of God and I shall bring down my wrath on you if I don't get my way."
- **Delusions of guilt:** Belief that one is guilty or responsible for something. Example: "I am responsible for all the world's wars."
- **Somatic delusions:** Belief that one has a certain illness or health condition. Example: A patient believing she is pregnant despite negative pregnancy tests and ultrasounds.

PERCEPTUAL DISTURBANCES

- **Illusion:** Misinterpretation of an existing sensory stimulus (such as mistaking a shadow for an evil spirit).
- **Hallucination:** Sensory perception without an actual external stimulus.
  - **Auditory:** The most common modality experienced by patients with schizophrenia.
  - **Visual:** Occurs in schizophrenia and other psychotic disorders, but less common. May accompany drug intoxication, drug and alcohol withdrawal, or delirium.
  - **Olfactory:** Usually an aura associated with epilepsy.
  - **Tactile:** Usually secondary to drug intoxication (e.g., cocaine or psychostimulants) or alcohol withdrawal.

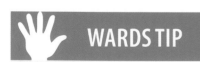

WARDS TIP

Auditory hallucinations that directly tell the patient to perform certain acts are called *command hallucinations*.

DIFFERENTIAL DIAGNOSIS OF PSYCHOSIS

- Psychotic disorder due to another medical condition.
- Substance/Medication-induced psychotic disorder.
- Delirium/Major neurocognitive disorder (dementia).
- Bipolar disorder, manic/mixed episode.
- Major depressive disorder with psychotic features.
- Brief psychotic disorder.
- Schizophrenia.
- Schizophreniform disorder.
- Schizoaffective disorder.
- Delusional disorder.

PSYCHOTIC DISORDER DUE TO ANOTHER MEDICAL CONDITION

Other Medical causes of psychosis include:

1. *Central nervous system (CNS) disease* (cerebrovascular disease, multiple sclerosis, neoplasm, Alzheimer disease, Parkinson disease, Huntington disease, tertiary syphilis, epilepsy [often temporal lobe], encephalitis, prion disease, neurosarcoidosis, AIDS).
2. *Endocrinopathies* (Addison/Cushing disease, hyper/hypothyroidism, hyper/hypocalcemia, hypopituitarism).
3. *Nutritional/Vitamin deficiency states* (B12, folate, niacin).
4. *Other* (connective tissue disease [systemic lupus erythematosus, temporal arteritis], porphyria).

DSM-5 **criteria** for psychotic disorder due to another medical condition include:

- Prominent hallucinations or delusions.
- Symptoms do not occur only during an episode of delirium.
- Evidence from history, physical, or lab data to support another medical cause (i.e., not a primary psychiatric disorder).

SUBSTANCE/MEDICATION-INDUCED PSYCHOTIC DISORDER

Prescription medications that may cause psychosis in some patients include anesthetics, antimicrobials, corticosteroids, antiparkinsonian agents, anticonvulsants, antihistamines, anticholinergics, antihypertensives, nonsteroidal anti-inflammatory drugs (NSAIDs), digitalis, methylphenidate, and chemotherapeutic agents. Substances such as alcohol, cocaine, hallucinogens (LSD, ecstasy), cannabis, benzodiazepines, barbiturates, inhalants, and phencyclidine (PCP) can cause psychosis, either during intoxication or withdrawal.

DSM-5 **Criteria**

- Hallucinations and/or delusions.
- Symptoms do not occur only during episode of delirium.
- Evidence from history, physical, or lab data to support a medication or substance-induced cause.
- Disturbance is not better accounted for by a psychotic disorder that is not substance/medication-induced.

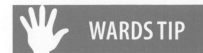

WARDS TIP

It's important to be able to distinguish between a delusion, illusion, and hallucination. A delusion is a fixed, false belief, an illusion is a misinterpretation of an external stimulus, and a hallucination is perception in the absence of an external stimulus.

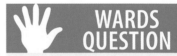

WARDS QUESTION

Q: What is the most likely etiology in an elderly, medically ill patient presenting with the new onset of psychotic symptoms?
A: Delirium.

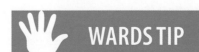

WARDS TIP

To make the diagnosis of schizophrenia, a patient must have symptoms of the disease for at least 6 months.

Schizophrenia

 A 24-year-old male graduate student without prior medical or psychiatric history is reported by his mother to have been very anxious over the past 9 months, with increasing concern that people are watching him. He now claims to "hear voices" telling him what must be done to "fix the country." *Important workup?* Comprehensive metabolic panel, urine drug screen, thyroid-stimulating hormone (TSH), HIV testing. Consider brain imaging. *Likely diagnosis? If workup is unremarkable,* schizophrenia. *Next step?* Antipsychotics.

Schizophrenia is a psychiatric disorder characterized by a constellation of abnormalities in thinking, emotion, and behavior. There is no single symptom that is pathognomonic, and there is a heterogeneous clinical presentation. Schizophrenia is typically chronic, with significant psychosocial and medical consequences to the patient.

POSITIVE, NEGATIVE, AND COGNITIVE SYMPTOMS

In general, the symptoms of schizophrenia are broken up into three categories:

- **Positive symptoms:** Hallucinations, delusions, bizarre behavior, disorganized speech. These tend to respond more robustly to antipsychotic medications.
- **Negative symptoms:** Flat or blunted affect, anhedonia, apathy, alogia, and lack of interest in socialization. These symptoms are comparatively more often treatment resistant and contribute significantly to the social isolation and impaired function of schizophrenic patients.
- **Cognitive symptoms:** Impairments in attention, executive function, and working memory. These symptoms may **lead to** poor work and school performance.

THREE PHASES

Symptoms of schizophrenia often present in the following three phases:
1. **Prodromal:** Decline in functioning that precedes the first psychotic episode. The patient may become socially withdrawn and irritable. They may have physical complaints, declining school/work performance, and/or newfound interest in religion or the occult.
2. **Psychotic:** Perceptual disturbances, delusions, and disordered thought process/content.
3. **Residual:** Occurs following an episode of active psychosis. It is marked by mild hallucinations or delusions, social withdrawal, and negative symptoms.

DIAGNOSIS OF SCHIZOPHRENIA

DSM-5 Criteria

- *Two or more of the following must be present for at least 1 month:*
  1. Delusions.
  2. Hallucinations.
  3. Disorganized speech.
  4. Grossly disorganized or catatonic behavior.
  5. Negative symptoms.

KEY FACT

Think of positive symptoms as things that are ADDED onto normal behavior. Think of negative symptoms as things that are SUB-TRACTED or missing from normal behavior.

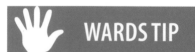

WARDS TIP

Stereotyped movement, bizarre posturing, and muscle rigidity are examples of catatonia, a syndrome which can be seen in schizophrenia, depression, bipolar disorder, and other psychiatric conditions.

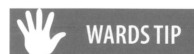

WARDS TIP

The 5 A's of schizophrenia (negative symptoms):

1. Anhedonia
2. Affect (flat)
3. Alogia (poverty of speech)
4. Avolition (apathy)
5. Attention (poor)

Note: At least one must be **1**, **2**, or **3**.

- Must cause significant social, occupational, or functional (self-care) deterioration.
- Duration of illness for at least 6 months (including prodromal or residual periods in which the above full criteria may not be met).
- Symptoms not due to effects of a substance or another medical condition.

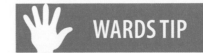

WARDS TIP

- Echolalia—Repeats words or phrases
- EchoPRAxia—Mimics behavior (PRActices behavior)

 Mr. T is a 21-year-old man who is brought to the ER by his mother after he began talking about "aliens" who were trying to steal his soul. He reports that aliens leave messages for him by arranging sticks outside his home and sometimes send thoughts into his mind. On exam, he is guarded and often stops talking while in the middle of expressing a thought. Mr. T appears anxious and frequently scans the room for aliens, which he thinks may have followed him to the hospital. He denies any plan to harm himself, but admits that the aliens sometimes want him to throw himself in front of a car, "as this will change the systems that belong under us."

The patient's mother reports that he began expressing these ideas a few months ago, but they have become more severe in the last few weeks. She reports that during the past year, he has become isolated from his peers, frequently talks to himself, and has stopped going to community college. He has also spent most of his time reading science fiction books and creating devices that will prevent aliens from hurting him. She reports that she is concerned because the patient's father, who left while the patient was a child, exhibited similar symptoms many years ago and has spent most of his life in psychiatric hospitals.

What is the patient's most likely diagnosis? What differential diagnoses should be considered?

Mr. T's most likely diagnosis is schizophrenia. He exhibits delusional ideas that are bizarre and paranoid in nature. He also reports the presence of frequent auditory hallucinations and disturbances in thought process that include thought blocking. Although the patient's mother reports that his psychotic symptoms began "a few months ago," the patient has exhibited social and occupational dysfunction during the last year. Mr. T quit school, became isolated, and has been responding to internal stimuli since that time. In addition, his father appears to also suffer from a psychotic disorder. In this case, it appears that the disorder has been present for more than 6 months. However, if this is unclear, the diagnosis of schizophreniform disorder should be made instead.

The differential diagnosis should also include schizoaffective disorder, medication/substance-induced psychotic disorder, psychotic disorder due to another medical condition, and mood disorder with psychotic features.

What would be appropriate steps in the acute management of this patient?

Treatment should include inpatient hospitalization in order to provide a safe environment, with monitoring of suicidal ideation secondary to his psychosis. Routine laboratory tests, including a urine or serum drug screen, should be undertaken. The patient should begin treatment with antipsychotic medication while closely being monitored for potential side effects.

PSYCHIATRIC EXAM OF PATIENTS WITH SCHIZOPHRENIA

The *typical* findings in patients with schizophrenia include:

- Disheveled appearance.
- Flat affect.

KEY FACT

Brief psychotic disorder lasts for <1 month. Schizophreniform disorder can last between 1 and 6 months. Schizophrenia lasts for >6 months.

- Disorganized thought process.
- Intact procedural memory and orientation.
- Auditory hallucinations.
- Paranoid delusions.
- Ideas of reference.
- Lack of insight into their disease.

Keep in mind that schizophrenia can have a very heterogeneous presentation—patients may have schizophrenia without a disheveled appearance or clear negative symptoms.

EPIDEMIOLOGY

- Schizophrenia affects approximately 0.3–0.7% of people over their lifetime.
- Men and women are equally affected but have different presentations and outcomes:
  - Men tend to present in early to mid-20s.
  - Women present in late 20s.
  - Men tend to have more negative symptoms and poorer outcome compared to women.
- Schizophrenia rarely presents before age 15 or after age 55.
- There is a strong genetic predisposition:
  - Fifty percent concordance rate among monozygotic twins.
  - Forty percent risk of inheritance if both parents have schizophrenia.
  - Twelve percent risk if one first-degree relative is affected.
- Substance use is comorbid in many patients with schizophrenia. The most commonly abused substance is nicotine (>50%), followed by alcohol, cannabis, and cocaine.
- Post-psychotic depression is the phenomenon of schizophrenic patients developing a major depressive episode after resolution of their psychotic symptoms.

DOWNWARD DRIFT

Lower socioeconomic groups have higher rates of schizophrenia. This may be due to the **downward drift hypothesis**, which postulates that people suffering from schizophrenia are unable to function well in society and hence end up in lower socioeconomic groups. Many homeless people in urban areas suffer from schizophrenia.

PATHOPHYSIOLOGY OF SCHIZOPHRENIA: THE DOPAMINE HYPOTHESIS

Though the exact cause of schizophrenia is not known, it appears to be partly related to increased dopamine activity in certain neuronal tracts. Evidence to support this hypothesis is that most antipsychotics successful in treating schizophrenia are dopamine receptor antagonists. In addition, cocaine and amphetamines increase dopamine activity and can cause schizophrenia-like symptoms.

Theorized Dopamine Pathways Affected in Schizophrenia

- *Prefrontal cortical:* Inadequate dopaminergic activity; responsible for negative symptoms.
- *Mesolimbic:* Excessive dopaminergic activity; responsible for positive symptoms.

KEY FACT

Schizophrenia is more prevalent in lower socioeconomic groups likely due to "downward drift" (many patients face barriers to higher education, regular employment, and other resources, so they tend to drift downward socioeconomically).

Other Important Dopamine Pathways Affected by Antipsychotics

- *Tuberoinfundibular:* Blocked by antipsychotics, causing hyperprolactinemia, which may lead to gynecomastia, galactorrhea, sexual dysfunction, and menstrual irregularities.
- *Nigrostriatal:* Blocked by antipsychotics, causing Parkinsonism/extrapyramidal side effects such as tremor, rigidity, slurred speech, akathisia, dystonia, and other abnormal movements.

OTHER NEUROTRANSMITTER ABNORMALITIES IMPLICATED IN SCHIZOPHRENIA

- **Elevated serotonin:** Some of the second-generation (atypical) antipsychotics (e.g., risperidone and clozapine) antagonize serotonin and weakly antagonize dopamine.
- **Elevated norepinephrine:** Long-term use of antipsychotics has been shown to decrease activity of noradrenergic neurons.
- **Low gamma-aminobutyric acid (GABA):** There is lower expression of the enzyme necessary to create GABA in the hippocampus of patients with schizophrenia.
- **Low levels of glutamate receptors:** Patients with schizophrenia have fewer NMDA receptors; this corresponds to the psychotic symptoms observed with NMDA antagonists like ketamine.

PROGNOSTIC FACTORS

Even with medication, 40–60% of patients remain significantly impaired after their diagnosis, while only 20–30% function fairly well in society. About 20% of patients with schizophrenia attempt suicide and many more experience suicidal ideation. Several factors are associated with a better or worse prognosis:

Associated with Better Prognosis

- Later onset.
- Good social support.
- Positive symptoms.
- Mood symptoms.
- Acute onset.
- Female gender.
- Few relapses.
- Good premorbid functioning.

Associated with Worse Prognosis

- Early onset.
- Poor social support.
- Negative symptoms.
- Family history.
- Gradual onset.
- Male gender.
- Many relapses.

KEY FACT

Akathisia is an unpleasant, subjective sense of restlessness and need to move, often manifested by the inability to sit still. Severe akathisia can be a risk factor for suicide.

WARDS QUESTION

Q: What are the most appropriate treatments for akathisia?
A: Tapering down antipsychotic medication, beta-blockers such as propranolol, or benzodiazepines.

KEY FACT

The lifetime prevalence of schizophrenia is 0.3–0.7%.

KEY FACT

Schizophrenia has a large genetic component. If one identical twin has schizophrenia, the risk of the other identical twin having schizophrenia is 50%. A biological child of a schizophrenic person has a higher chance of developing schizophrenia, even if adopted into a family without schizophrenia.

KEY FACT

Computed tomography (CT) and magnetic resonance imaging (MRI) scans of patients with schizophrenia may show enlargement of the ventricles, diffuse cortical atrophy, and reduced brain volume.

KEY FACT

Schizophrenia often involves neologisms. A neologism is a newly coined word or expression that has meaning only to the person who uses it.

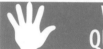

WARDS QUESTION

Q: What is the typical age of onset for schizophrenia?
A: For men, 15–25. For women, 15–30, with a second (smaller) peak incidence in the late 40s.

WARDS TIP

First-generation antipsychotic medications are referred to as typical or conventional antipsychotics (often called neuroleptics). Second-generation antipsychotic medications are referred to as atypical antipsychotics.

- Poor premorbid functioning (social isolation, etc.).
- Comorbid substance use.

TREATMENT

A multimodal approach is the most effective, and therapy must be tailored to the needs of the specific patient. **Pharmacologic** treatment consists primarily of antipsychotic medications. (For more detail, see Chapter 18, "Psychopharmacology.")

- **First-generation (or typical) antipsychotic medications**
  (e.g., *chlorpromazine, fluphenazine, haloperidol, perphenazine*):
  - Primarily dopamine (mostly D2) antagonists.
  - Treat positive symptoms with minimal impact on negative symptoms.
  - Side effects include extrapyramidal symptoms, neuroleptic malignant syndrome, and tardive dyskinesia (see below).
- **Second-generation (or atypical) antipsychotic medications**
  (e.g., *aripiprazole, asenapine, clozapine, iloperidone, lurasidone, olanzapine, quetiapine, risperidone, ziprasidone*):
  - These antagonize serotonin receptors (5-HT2) as well as dopamine (D4>D2) receptors.
  - Research has not shown a significant difference between first- and second-generation antipsychotics in efficacy. The selection requires the weighing of benefits and risks in individual clinical cases.
  - Lower incidence of extrapyramidal side effects, but higher risk of metabolic syndrome.
  - Medications should be taken for at least 4 weeks before efficacy is determined.
  - Clozapine is reserved for patients who have failed multiple antipsychotic trials due to its risk of agranulocytosis.

Behavioral therapy attempts to improve patients' ability to function in society. Patients are helped through a variety of methods to improve their social skills, become self-sufficient, and minimize disruptive behaviors. **Family therapy** and **group therapy** are also useful adjuncts.

Important Side Effects and Sequelae of Antipsychotic Medications
Side effects of antipsychotic medications include:
1. Extrapyramidal symptoms (especially with the use of high-potency first-generation antipsychotics):
   - Dystonia (spasms") of face, neck, and tongue.
   - Parkinsonism (resting tremor, rigidity, bradykinesia).
   - Akathisia (feeling of restlessness).
   - *Treatment:* Anticholinergics (benztropine, diphenhydramine), benzodiazepines/beta-blockers (specifically for akathisia).
2. Anticholinergic symptoms (especially low-potency first-generation antipsychotics and atypical antipsychotics): Dry mouth, constipation, blurred vision, hyperthermia.
   Treatment: As per symptom (eye drops, stool softeners, etc.).
3. Metabolic syndrome (second-generation antipsychotics): A constellation of conditions— **elevated** blood pressure, **elevated** blood sugar levels, excess

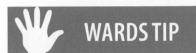

body fat around the waist, abnormal cholesterol levels—that occur together, **increasing** the risk for cardiovascular disease, stroke, and type 2 diabetes.

Treatment: Consider switching to a first-generation antipsychotic or a more "weight-neutral" second-generation antipsychotic such as aripiprazole or ziprasidone. Consider metformin if the patient is not already on it. Monitor lipids and blood glucose measurements. Refer the patient to primary care for appropriate treatment of hyperlipidemia, diabetes, etc. Encourage appropriate diet, exercise, and smoking cessation.

4. Tardive dyskinesia (more likely with first-generation antipsychotics): Choreoathetoid movements, usually seen in the face, tongue, and head.

   Treatment: Discontinue or reduce the medication and consider substituting an atypical antipsychotic (if appropriate). VMAT-2 inhibitors such as valbenazine, benzodiazepines, Botox, and vitamin E may be used. The movements may persist despite withdrawal of the drug. Although less common, atypical antipsychotics can also cause tardive dyskinesia.

5. Neuroleptic malignant syndrome (NMS) (typically high-potency first-generation antipsychotics):

   - Change in mental status, autonomic instability (high fever, labile blood pressure, tachycardia, tachypnea, diaphoresis), "lead pipe" rigidity, elevated creatine kinase (CK) levels, leukocytosis, and metabolic acidosis. Reflexes are decreased.

   - NMS is a **medical emergency** that requires prompt withdrawal of all antipsychotic medications and immediate medical assessment and treatment.

   - May be observed in any patient being treated with any antipsychotic (including second generation) medications at any time, but is more frequently associated with the initiation of treatment and at higher IV/IM dosing of high-potency neuroleptics.

   - Patients with a history of prior neuroleptic malignant syndrome are at increased risk of recurrent episodes when retrialed with antipsychotic agents.

6. Prolonged QTc interval and other electrocardiogram changes, hyperprolactinemia (gynecomastia, galactorrhea, amenorrhea, diminished libido, and impotence), hematologic effects (agranulocytosis may occur with *clozapine*, requiring frequent blood draws when this medication is used), ophthalmologic conditions (*thioridazine* may cause irreversible retinal pigmentation at high doses; deposits in lens and cornea may occur with *chlorpromazine*), dermatologic conditions (such as rashes and photosensitivity).

Schizophreniform Disorder

Diagnosis and DSM-5 Criteria

The diagnosis of schizophreniform disorder is made using the same *DSM-5* criteria as schizophrenia. The only difference is that in schizophreniform disorder the symptoms have lasted between 1 and 6 months, whereas in schizophrenia the symptoms must be present for >6 months.

Prognosis

One-third of patients recover completely; two-thirds progress to schizoaffective disorder or schizophrenia.

Treatment

Hospitalization (if necessary), 6-month course of antipsychotics, and supportive psychotherapy.

WARDS TIP

Patients who are treated with *first-generation* (typical) antipsychotic medication need to be closely monitored for extrapyramidal symptoms, such as acute dystonia and tardive dyskinesia.

WARDS TIP

Patients with schizophrenia who are treated with *second-generation* (atypical) antipsychotic medications need a careful medical evaluation for metabolic syndrome. This includes checking weight, body mass index (BMI), fasting blood glucose or HbA1c, lipid assessment, and blood pressure.

KEY FACT

High-potency antipsychotics (such as haloperidol and fluphenazine) have a higher incidence of extrapyramidal side effects, while *low-potency* antipsychotics (such as chlorpromazine) have primarily anticholinergic and antiadrenergic side effects.

WARDS QUESTION

Q: What antipsychotic medications are available as long-acting injectables?
A: First generation: haloperidol, fluphenazine. Second generation: risperidone, paliperidone, aripiprazole, olanzapine.

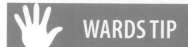

WARDS TIP

Tardive dyskinesia occurs most often in older women after at least 6 months of medication. A small percentage of patients will experience spontaneous remission, so discontinuation of the agent should be considered if clinically appropriate.

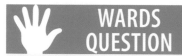

WARDS TIP

The cumulative risk of developing tardive dyskinesia from antipsychotics (particularly first generation) is 5% per year.

WARDS QUESTION

Q: Which antipsychotic has been shown to reduce suicidality in patients with schizophrenia?
A: Clozapine.

WARDS TIP

Clozapine is typically considered for treating schizophrenia when a patient fails both typical and other atypical antipsychotics. It is a very effective medication, but can cause agranulocytosis; therefore, patients' white blood cell and absolute neutrophil counts must be monitored regularly. Clozapine also has black box warnings for orthostatic hypotension, seizures, and cardiomyopathy. Other common side effects include sedation, excessive drooling, and severe constipation.

Schizoaffective Disorder

Diagnosis and DSM-5 Criteria

The diagnosis of schizoaffective disorder is made in patients who:

- Meet criteria for either a major depressive or manic episode during which psychotic symptoms consistent with schizophrenia are also met.
- Have delusions or hallucinations for 2 weeks in the absence of mood disorder symptoms (this criterion is necessary to differentiate schizoaffective disorder from a mood disorder with psychotic features).
- Have mood symptoms for a majority of the psychotic illness.
- Have symptoms not due to the effects of a substance (drug or medication) or another medical condition.

Prognosis

Worse with poor premorbid adjustment, slow onset, early onset, predominance of psychotic symptoms, long course, and family history of schizophrenia.

Treatment

- Hospitalization (if necessary) and supportive psychotherapy.
- Medical therapy: Antipsychotics (second-generation medications may target both psychotic and mood symptoms); mood stabilizers, antidepressants, or electroconvulsive therapy (ECT) may be indicated for treatment of mood symptoms.

Brief Psychotic Disorder

Diagnosis and DSM-5 Criteria

Patient with psychotic symptoms as in schizophrenia; however, the symptoms last from 1 day to 1 month, and there must be eventual full return to premorbid level of functioning. Symptoms must not be due to the effects of a substance (drug or medication) or another medical condition. This is a rare diagnosis, much less common than schizophrenia. It may be seen in reaction to extreme stress such as bereavement and sexual assault.

Prognosis

High rates of relapse, but almost all completely recover.

Treatment

Brief hospitalization (usually required for workup, safety, and stabilization), supportive therapy, course of antipsychotics for psychosis, and/or benzodiazepines for agitation.

Delusional Disorder

Delusional disorder occurs more often in middle-aged or older patients (after age 40). Immigrants, the hearing impaired, and those with a family history of schizophrenia are at increased risk.

Diagnosis and DSM-5 Criteria

To be diagnosed with delusional disorder, the following criteria must be met:

- One or more delusions for at least 1 month.
- Does not meet criteria for schizophrenia.

TABLE 3-1. Schizophrenia versus Delusional Disorder	
Schizophrenia	**Delusional Disorder**

▪ Bizarre or nonbizarre delusions
▪ Daily functioning significantly impaired
▪ Must have two or more of the following:
  ▪ Delusions
  ▪ Hallucinations
  ▪ Disorganized speech
  ▪ Disorganized behavior
  ▪ Negative symptoms
	▪ Usually nonbizarre delusions
	▪ Daily functioning not significantly impaired
	▪ Does not meet the criteria for schizophrenia, as described in the left column

- Functioning in life not significantly impaired, and behavior not obviously bizarre.
- While delusions may be present in both delusional disorder and schizophrenia, there are important differences (see Table 3-1).

Types of Delusions
Patients are further categorized based on the types of delusions they experience:

- **Erotomanic type:** Delusion that another person is in love with the individual.
- **Grandiose type:** Delusions of having great talent.
- **Somatic type:** Physical delusions.
- **Persecutory type:** Delusions of being persecuted.
- **Jealous type:** Delusions of unfaithfulness.
- **Mixed type:** More than one of the above.
- **Unspecified type:** Not a specific type as described above.

Prognosis
Better than schizophrenia with treatment:

- >50%: Full recovery.
- >20%: Decrease in symptoms.
- <20%: No change.

Treatment
Difficult to treat, especially given the lack of insight and impairment. Antipsychotic medications are recommended despite somewhat limited evidence. Supportive therapy is often helpful.

Culture-Specific Psychoses

The following are examples of psychotic disorders seen within certain cultures:

	Psychotic Manifestation	Culture
Koro	Intense anxiety that the penis will recede into the body, possibly leading to death.	Southeast Asia (e.g., Singapore)
Amok	Sudden unprovoked outbursts of violence, often followed by suicide.	Malaysia
Brain fag	Headache, fatigue, eye pain, cognitive difficulties, and other somatic disturbances in male students.	Africa

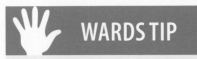

WARDS TIP

If a schizophrenia presentation has not been present for 6 months, think *schizophreniform disorder*.

KEY FACT

Patients with borderline personality disorder may have transient, stress-related psychotic experiences. These are considered part of their underlying personality disorder and are not diagnosed as a brief psychotic disorder.

Comparing Time Courses and Prognoses of Psychotic Disorders

Time Course

- <1 month—Brief psychotic disorder.
- 1–6 months—Schizophreniform disorder.
- >6 months—Schizophrenia.

Prognosis from Best to Worst

Mood disorder with psychotic features > schizoaffective disorder > schizophreniform disorder > schizophrenia.

QUICK AND EASY DISTINGUISHING FEATURES

- **Schizophrenia:** Lifelong psychotic disorder.
- **Schizophreniform:** Schizophrenia for >1 and <6 months.
- **Schizoaffective:** Distinct mood episodes with psychosis persisting between mood episodes.
- **Schizotypal** (personality disorder): Paranoid, odd or magical beliefs, eccentric, lack of friends, social anxiety. Criteria for overt psychosis are not met.
- **Schizoid** (personality disorder): Solitary activities, lack of enjoyment from social interactions, no psychosis.

KEY FACT

SchizophreniFORM = the FORMation of a schizophrenic, but not quite there (i.e., <6 months).

CHAPTER 4

MOOD DISORDERS

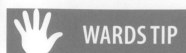

WARDS TIP

Major depressive episodes can be present in major depressive disorder, persistent depressive disorder (dysthymia), bipolar I/II disorder, and schizoaffective disorder.

WARDS TIP

When patients have delusions and hallucinations due to underlying mood disorders, they are usually mood congruent. For example, depression causes psychotic themes of paranoia and worthlessness, and mania causes psychotic themes of grandiosity and invincibility.

KEY FACT

Symptoms of major depression—SIG E. CAPS (Prescribe Energy Capsules)

Sleep

Interest

Guilt

Energy

Concentration

Appetite

Psychomotor activity

Suicidal ideation

Concepts in Mood Disorders

A **mood** is a description of one's internal emotional state. Both external and internal stimuli can trigger moods, which may be labeled as sad, happy, angry, irritable, and so on. It is normal to have a wide range of moods and to have a sense of control over one's moods.

Patients with mood *disorders* (also called affective disorders) experience an abnormal range of moods and lose some level of control over them. Distress may be caused by the severity of their moods and the resulting impairment in social and occupational functioning.

Mood Disorders versus Mood Episodes

- **Mood episodes** are distinct periods of time in which some abnormal mood is present. They include depression, mania, and hypomania.
- **Mood disorders** are defined by their patterns of mood episodes. They include major depressive disorder (MDD), bipolar I disorder, bipolar II disorder, persistent depressive disorder, and cyclothymic disorder. Some may have psychotic features (delusions or hallucinations).

Mood Episodes

MAJOR DEPRESSIVE EPISODE (MDE)

Must have at least five of the following symptoms (must include either number 1 or 2) for at least a 2-week period:

1. Depressed mood most of the time.
2. Anhedonia (loss of interest in pleasurable activities).
3. Change in appetite or weight ($\uparrow$ or $\downarrow$).
4. Feelings of worthlessness or excessive guilt.
5. Insomnia or hypersomnia.
6. Diminished concentration.
7. Psychomotor agitation or retardation (i.e., restlessness or slowness).
8. Fatigue or loss of energy.
9. Recurrent thoughts of death or suicide.

Symptoms must not be attributable to the effects of a substance (drug or medication) or another medical condition, and they must cause clinically significant distress or social/occupational impairment.

MANIC EPISODE

A distinct period of abnormally and persistently elevated, expansive, or irritable mood, and abnormally and persistently increased goal-directed activity or energy, lasting at least 1 week (or any duration if hospitalization is necessary), and including at least three of the following (four if the mood is only irritable):

1. Distractibility.
2. Inflated self-esteem or grandiosity.
3. $\uparrow$ in goal-directed activity (socially, at work, or sexually) or psychomotor agitation.

4. ↓ need for sleep.
5. Flight of ideas or racing thoughts.
6. More talkative than usual or *pressured speech* (rapid and uninterruptible).
7. Excessive involvement in pleasurable activities that have a high risk of negative consequences (e.g., shopping sprees, sexual indiscretions).

Symptoms must not be attributable to the effects of a substance (drug or medication) or another medical condition, and they must cause clinically significant distress or social/occupational impairment. Greater than 50% of patients with manic episodes have psychotic symptoms.

HYPOMANIC EPISODE

A hypomanic episode is a distinct period of abnormally and persistently elevated, expansive, or irritable mood, and abnormally and persistently increased goal-directed activity or energy, lasting at least 4 consecutive days, that includes at least three of the symptoms listed for the manic episode criteria (four if mood is only irritable). There are significant differences between mania and hypomania (see below).

DIFFERENCES BETWEEN MANIC AND HYPOMANIC EPISODES

Mania	Hypomania
Lasts at least 7 days	Lasts at least 4 days
Causes severe impairment in social or occupational functioning	No marked impairment in social or occupational functioning
May necessitate hospitalization to prevent harm to self or others	Does not require hospitalization
May have psychotic features	No psychotic features

MIXED FEATURES

Criteria are met for a manic or hypomanic episode and at least three symptoms of a MDE are present for the majority of the time. These criteria must be present nearly every day for at least 1 week.

Mood Disorders

Mood disorders often have chronic courses that are marked by relapses *with relatively normal functioning between episodes, which is a key factor in distinguishing a mood disorder from other chronic psychiatric disorders such as schizophrenia.* Like most psychiatric diagnoses, mood episodes may be caused by another medical condition or drug (prescribed or illicit). Therefore, always investigate medical or substance-induced causes (see below) before diagnosing a primary mood disorder.

DIFFERENTIAL DIAGNOSIS OF MOOD DISORDERS DUE TO OTHER MEDICAL CONDITIONS

Medical Causes of a Depressive Episode	Medical Causes of a Manic Episode
Cerebrovascular disease (stroke, myocardial infarction)	Metabolic (hyperthyroidism)
Endocrinopathies (diabetes mellitus, Cushing syndrome, Addison disease, hypoglycemia, hyper/hypothyroidism, hyper/hypocalcemia)	Neurological disorders (temporal lobe seizures, multiple sclerosis)

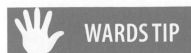

WARDS TIP

A suicide risk assessment should include evaluating current or recent suicidal ideation (including wishing to be dead, thinking of methods, planning, or having intent) and should assess frequency, duration, and intensity of these thoughts.

Suicide Risk Factors:
SAD PERSONS
S: Male sex
A: <19 or >45 years
D: Depression
P: Previous attempt
E: Excess alcohol or substance use
R: Rational thinking loss
S: Social supports lacking
O: Organized plan
N: No spouse
S: Sickness

KEY FACT

Symptoms of mania—**DIG FAST**
Distractibility
Insomnia/Impulsive behavior
Grandiosity
Flight of ideas/Racing thoughts
Activity/Agitation
Speech (pressured)
Thoughtlessness

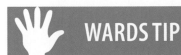

WARDS TIP

A manic episode is a psychiatric emergency; severely impaired judgment and impulsivity can make a patient dangerous to self and others.

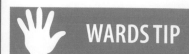

Irritability is often the predominant mood state in mood disorders with mixed features. Patients with mixed features have a poorer response to lithium. Anticonvulsants such as valproic acid may be more helpful.

KEY FACT

Patients with cardiovascular disease or strokes are at a significant risk for developing depression, and this is associated with a poorer outcome overall.

KEY FACT

Depression is common in patients with pancreatic cancer.

Parkinson disease	Neoplasms
Viral illnesses (e.g., mononucleosis)	HIV infection
Carcinoid syndrome	
Cancer (especially lymphoma and pancreatic carcinoma)	
Collagen vascular disease (e.g., systemic lupus erythematosus)	

SUBSTANCE/MEDICATION-INDUCED MOOD DISORDERS

Substance/Medication-Induced Depressive Disorder	Substance/Medication-Induced Bipolar Disorder
EtOH	Antidepressants
Antihypertensives	Sympathomimetics
Barbiturates	Dopamine
Corticosteroids	Corticosteroids
Levodopa	Levodopa
Sedative-hypnotics	Bronchodilators
Anticonvulsants	Cocaine
Antipsychotics	Amphetamines
Diuretics	
Sulfonamides	
Opiates	
Withdrawal from stimulants (e.g., cocaine, amphetamines)	

 Ms. Cruz is a 28-year-old sales clerk who arrives at your outpatient clinic complaining of sadness after her boyfriend of 6 months ended their relationship 1 month ago. She describes a history of failed romantic relationships, and says, "I don't do well with breakups." Ms. Cruz reports that, although she has no prior psychiatric treatment, she was urged by her employer to seek therapy. Ms. Cruz has arrived late to work on several occasions because of oversleeping. She also has difficulty in getting out of bed stating, "It's difficult to walk; it's like my legs weigh a ton." She feels fatigued during the day despite spending over 12 hours in bed, and is concerned that she might be suffering from a serious medical condition. She denies any significant changes in appetite or weight since these symptoms began.

Ms. Cruz reports that, although she has not missed workdays, she has difficulty concentrating and has become tearful in front of clients while worrying about not finding a significant other. She feels tremendous guilt over "not being good enough to get married," and says that her close friends are concerned because she has been spending her weekends in bed and not answering their calls. Although during your evaluation Ms. Cruz appears tearful, she brightens up when talking about her newborn nephew and her plans to visit a college friend next summer. Ms. Cruz denies suicidal ideation.

What is Ms. Cruz's diagnosis?

Ms. Cruz's diagnosis is MDD with atypical features. She complains of sadness, fatigue, poor concentration, hypersomnia, feelings of guilt, anhedonia, and impairment in her social and occupational functioning. The atypical features specifier is given in this case as she exhibited mood reactivity (mood brightens in response to positive events) when talking about her nephew and visiting her friend, and complained of a heavy feeling in her legs (leaden paralysis) and hypersomnia. It is also important to explore Ms. Cruz's history of "not doing well with breakups," as this could be indicative of a long pattern of interpersonal rejection sensitivity. Although it is common for patients who suffer from atypical depression to report an ↑ in appetite, Ms. Cruz exhibits enough symptoms to fulfill atypical features criteria. Adjustment disorder should also be considered in the differential diagnosis.

What would be your pharmacological recommendation?

Ms. Cruz should be treated with an antidepressant medication. While monoamine oxidase inhibitors (MAOIs) such as phenelzine had traditionally been superior to tricyclic antidepressants (TCAs) in the treatment of MDD with atypical features, selective serotonin reuptake inhibitors (SSRIs) would be the first-line treatment given more favorable safety and side-effect profile. The combination of pharmacotherapy and psychotherapy has been shown to be more effective for treating mild-to-moderate MDD than either treatment alone.

MAJOR DEPRESSIVE DISORDER (MDD)

MDD is marked by episodes of depressed mood associated with loss of interest in daily activities. Patients may not acknowledge their depressed mood or may express vague, somatic complaints (fatigue, headache, abdominal pain, muscle tension, etc.).

Diagnosis and DSM-5 Criteria

- At least one MDE (see above).
- No history of manic or hypomanic episode.

Epidemiology

- Lifetime prevalence: 12% worldwide.
- Onset at any age, but the age of onset peaks in the 20s.
- 1.5–2 times as prevalent in women than men during reproductive years.
- No ethnic or socioeconomic differences.
- Lifetime prevalence in the elderly: <10%.
- Depression can ↑ mortality for patients with other comorbidities such as diabetes, stroke, and cardiovascular disease.

Sleep Problems Associated with MDD

- Multiple awakenings.
- Initial and terminal insomnia (hard to fall asleep and early morning awakenings).
- Hypersomnia (excessive sleepiness) is less common.
- Rapid eye movement (REM) sleep shifted earlier in the night and for a greater duration, with reduced stages 3 and 4 (slow wave) sleep.
- Caution: Other medical conditions like obstructive sleep apnea (OSA) can cause sleep disturbances with associated changes in energy or mood that can mimic symptoms of depression.

Etiology

The precise cause of depression is unknown, but MDD is believed to be a heterogeneous disease, with biological, genetic, environmental, and psychosocial factors contributing.

- MDD is likely caused by neurotransmitter abnormalities in the brain. Evidence for this is the following: antidepressants exert their therapeutic effect by increasing catecholamines; ↓ cerebrospinal fluid (CSF) levels of

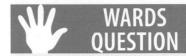

KEY FACT

Anhedonia is the inability to experience pleasure, and **apathy** is the inability to feel interested or motivated; both are a common finding in depression.

WARDS QUESTION

Q: What are the most common psychiatric disorders among those who commit suicide?
A: MDD and bipolar I disorder.

WARDS TIP

The two most common types of sleep disturbances associated with MDD are difficulty falling asleep and early morning awakenings.

The Hamilton Depression Rating Scale (HAM-D) measures the severity of depression and is used in research to assess the effectiveness of therapies. PHQ-9 is a depression screening form often used in the primary care setting.

KEY FACT

Loss of a parent before age 11 is associated with the later development of major depression.

KEY FACT

Most adults with depression do not see a mental health professional, but they often first present to a primary care physician for other reasons.

KEY FACT

Unfortunately only half of patients with MDD receive treatment.

5-hydroxyindolacetic acid (5-HIAA), the main metabolite of serotonin, have been found in depressed patients with impulsive and suicidal behavior.

■ Increased sensitivity of beta-adrenergic receptors in the brain has also been postulated in the pathogenesis of MDD.

■ **High cortisol:** Hyperactivity of hypothalamic-pituitary-adrenal axis, as shown by failure to suppress cortisol levels in the dexamethasone suppression test.

■ **Abnormal thyroid axis:** Thyroid disorders are associated with depressive symptoms.

■ Gamma-aminobutyric acid (GABA), glutamate, and endogenous opiates may additionally have a role.

■ **Psychosocial/Life events:** Multiple adverse childhood experiences (ACEs) are a risk factor for later developing MDD.

■ **Genetics:** First-degree relatives are two to four times more likely to have MDD. Concordance rate for monozygotic twins is <40%, and for dizygotic twins is 10–20%.

Course and Prognosis

■ Untreated, depressive episodes are self-limiting but last from 6 to 12 months. Generally, episodes occur more frequently as the disorder progresses. The risk of a subsequent MDE is 50–60% within the first 2 years after the first episode. Up to 15% of patients with MDD eventually commit suicide.

■ Approximately 60–70% of patients show a significant response to antidepressants. The gold standard for treatment of MDD is the combined use of both an antidepressant and psychotherapy, which produces a significantly ↑ response.

Treatment

Hospitalization

■ Indicated if the patient is at risk for suicide, homicide, or is unable to care for themselves.

Pharmacotherapy

■ **Antidepressant medications:**

• *Selective serotonin reuptake inhibitors (SSRIs):* Inhibit the reuptake of serotonin, thus increasing the amount of serotonin in the brain. Safer and better tolerated than other classes of antidepressants; side effects are mild but include headache, *gastrointestinal disturbance, sexual dysfunction*, and rebound anxiety. Examples are fluoxetine (Prozac®), escitalopram (Lexapro®), and sertraline (Zoloft®).

• *Serotonin-norepinephrine reuptake inhibitors (SNRIs):* Inhibit the reuptake of both serotonin and norepinephrine, thus increasing the level of both neurotransmitters in the brain. Includes venlafaxine (Effexor®) and duloxetine (Cymbalta®).

• *Other antidepressants:* Other agents commonly used to treat depression include the α2-adrenergic receptor antagonist mirtazapine (Remeron®), and the dopamine-norepinephrine reuptake inhibitor bupropion (Wellbutrin®).

• *Tricyclic antidepressants (TCAs):* Most lethal in overdose due to cardiac arrhythmias; side effects include sedation, weight gain, orthostatic hypotension, and anticholinergic effects. Can aggravate prolonged QTc syndrome.

- *Monoamine oxidase inhibitors (MAOIs):* Older medications rarely used for refractory depression; risk of *hypertensive crisis* when used with sympathomimetics or ingestion of tyramine-rich foods, such as wine, beer, aged cheeses, liver, and smoked meats (tyramine is an intermediate in the conversion of tyrosine to norepinephrine); risk of *serotonin syndrome* when used in combination with SSRIs. Most common side effect is orthostatic hypotension.
- *Novel agents:* Newer agents acting with unique mechanisms are available such as vilazodone (Viibryd) which has serotonin partial agonism, or vortioxetine (Trintilix) which interacts with additional serotonin receptors. Note: new medications can be prohibitively expensive until the generic form is available

■ **Adjunct medications:**

- Atypical (second-generation) antipsychotics along with antidepressants are first-line treatment in patients with MDD with psychotic features. In addition, they may also be prescribed in patients with treatment resistant/refractory MDD without psychotic features.
- Triiodothyronine (T3), levothyroxine (T4), and lithium have demonstrated some benefit when augmenting antidepressants in treatment refractory MDD.
- While stimulants (such as methylphenidate) may be used in certain patients (e.g., geriatric and terminally ill patients), the efficacy is limited and trials are small.

Psychotherapy

■ Cognitive-behavioral therapy (CBT), interpersonal psychotherapy, supportive therapy, psychodynamic psychotherapy, problem-solving therapy, and family/couples therapy have all demonstrated benefit in treating MDD.

- Among the major kinds of psychotherapy, there is no compelling evidence that one is superior to the rest. The choice is usually based on availability and patient preference.
- CBT and interpersonal psychotherapy are often selected as initial treatment because they have been the most widely studied.

■ May be used alone or in conjunction with pharmacotherapy.

■ Early dropout is common (as with pharmacotherapy). It is important to track patient adherence over time.

Electroconvulsive Therapy (ECT)

■ Indicated if the patient is unresponsive to pharmacotherapy, if patient cannot tolerate pharmacotherapy (pregnancy, etc.), or if rapid reduction of symptoms is desired (e.g., immediate suicide risk, refusal to eat/drink, catatonia).

■ ECT is extremely safe (primary risk is from anesthesia) and may be used alone or in combination with pharmacotherapy.

■ ECT is often performed by premedication with atropine, followed by general anesthesia (e.g., methohexital) and administration of a muscle relaxant (typically succinylcholine). A generalized seizure is then induced by passing a current of electricity across the brain (either bilateral or unilateral); the seizure should last between 30 and 60 seconds, and no longer than 90 seconds.

■ 6–12 treatments are administered over a 2- to 3-week period, but significant improvement is sometimes noted after the first several treatments. Some

WARDS TIP

MAOIs were considered particularly useful in the treatment of "atypical" depression; however, SSRIs remain first-line treatment for MDEs with atypical features.

WARDS QUESTION

Q: What is the most effective antidepressant medication and how quickly does it work?
A: All antidepressant medications are equally effective but differ in side-effect profiles. Medications take 4–6 weeks to reach peak efficacy.

WARDS QUESTION

Q: What are the hallmark symptoms of serotonin syndrome?
A: Autonomic instability, hyperthermia, hyperreflexia (including myoclonus), and seizures. Coma or death may result.

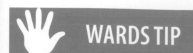

WARDS TIP

Adjunctive treatment is usually performed after multiple first-line treatment failures.

KEY FACT

The postpartum period conveys an elevated risk of depression in women.

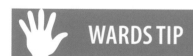

WARDS TIP

Triad for seasonal affective disorder:
- Irritability
- Carbohydrate craving
- Hypersomnia

KEY FACT

Bereavement is NOT a *DSM-5* diagnosis—if a patient meets criteria for MDD following the loss of a loved one, the diagnosis would be major depressive disorder.

patients require weekly or monthly maintenance ECT, though there is limited data on the efficacy of this.

- Retrograde and anterograde amnesia are common side effects, which usually resolve within 6 months.
- Other common but transient side effects: headache, nausea, muscle soreness.

SPECIFIERS FOR DEPRESSIVE DISORDERS

- **Melancholic features:** Present in approximately 25–30% of patients with a MDE and more likely in severely ill inpatients, including those with psychotic features. Characterized by *anhedonia*, early morning awakenings, depression worse in the morning, psychomotor disturbance, excessive guilt, and anorexia. For example, you would list the diagnosis as MDD with melancholic features.
- **Atypical features:** Characterized by hypersomnia, hyperphagia, reactive mood, leaden paralysis, and hypersensitivity to interpersonal rejection.
- **Mixed features:** Manic/hypomanic symptoms present during the majority of days during a MDE: elevated mood, grandiosity, talkativeness/pressured speech, flight of ideas/racing thoughts, increased energy/goal-directed activity, excessive involvement in dangerous activities, and decreased need for sleep.
- **Catatonia:** Features include catalepsy (immobility), purposeless motor activity, extreme negativism (resistance to instructions), staring, mutism, bizarre postures, and echolalia. Treatment is lorazepam (Ativan) though catatonia is especially responsive to ECT. (May also be applied to bipolar disorder.)
- **Psychotic features:** Characterized by the presence of delusions and/or hallucinations. Present in 24–53% of older, hospitalized patients with MDD.
- **Anxious distress:** Defined by feeling keyed up/tense, restless, difficulty concentrating, fears of something bad happening, and feelings of loss of control.
- **Peripartum onset:** Onset of MDD symptoms occurs during pregnancy or 4 weeks following delivery.
- **Seasonal pattern:** Temporal relationship between the onset of a MDE and particular time of the year (most commonly the winter but may occur in any season). Patients with fall-onset SAD (seasonal affective disorder or "winter depression") often respond to light therapy (a 10,000 lux white light for 30 minutes in the early morning).

BEREAVEMENT

Bereavement, also known as simple grief, is a normal reaction to a major loss, usually of a loved one, and it is not a mental illness. While symptoms are usually self-limited and only last for several months, if an individual meets criteria for a depressive episode, they would be diagnosed with MDD. Normal bereavement should not include gross psychotic symptoms, disorganization, or active suicidality.

BIPOLAR I DISORDER

Bipolar I disorder involves episodes of mania and of major depression; however, episodes of major depression are *not* required for the diagnosis. It is also known as **manic-depression**.

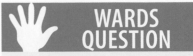

Diagnosis and DSM-5 Criteria

The only requirement for this diagnosis is the occurrence of a **manic episode** (5% of patients experience only manic episodes). Between manic episodes, there may be interspersed euthymia, MDEs, or hypomanic episodes, but none of these are required for the diagnosis. There is usually a return to baseline functioning in between mood episodes.

Epidemiology

- Lifetime prevalence: 1–2%.
- Women and men are equally affected.
- No ethnic differences seen; however, high-income countries have twice the rate of low-income countries (1.4% versus 0.7%).
- Onset usually before age 30, mean age of first mood episode is 18.
- Frequently misdiagnosed as unipolar depression and thereby inappropriately or inadequately treated.

Etiology

- Biological, environmental, psychosocial, and genetic factors are all important.
- First-degree relatives of patients with bipolar disorder are 10 times more likely to develop the illness.
- Concordance rates for monozygotic twins are 40–70%, and rates for dizygotic twins range from 5% to 25%.
- Bipolar I has the highest genetic link of all major psychiatric disorders.

Course and Prognosis

- Untreated manic episodes generally last several months.
- The course is usually chronic with relapses; as the disease progresses, episodes may occur more frequently.
- Ninety percent of individuals after one manic episode will have a repeat mood episode within 5 years.
- Bipolar disorder has a poorer prognosis than MDD: treatment refusal frequently occurs in patients with mania who enjoy their increased creativity and energy, and lack insight into the dangerousness of the illness.
- Maintenance treatment with mood stabilizing medications between episodes helps to ↓ the risk of relapse.
- 25–50% of people with bipolar disorder attempt suicide, and 10–15% die by suicide.

Treatment

- **Pharmacotherapy:**
  - Lithium remains the gold standard as a mood stabilizer; 50–70% treated with lithium show partial reduction of mania. The mechanism is unclear, but long-term use **reduces suicide risk**. Acute overdose can be fatal due to its narrow therapeutic index.
  - The anticonvulsants carbamazepine and valproic acid are also mood stabilizers. They are particularly useful for rapid cycling bipolar disorder and those with mixed features.
  - Atypical antipsychotics (e.g., risperidone, olanzapine, quetiapine, ziprasidone) are effective as both monotherapy and adjunct therapy for acute mania. In fact, many patients (especially with severe mania and/

WARDS QUESTION

Q: What is the most effective treatment for major depression with psychotic features?
A: Combination of an antidepressant **and** antipsychotic, **or** ECT.

WARDS QUESTION

Q: How is bipolar I disorder different from major depressive disorder?
A: Bipolar I disorder requires a manic episode.

WARDS QUESTION

Q: What is the first-line treatment for bipolar disorder?
A: Lithium, valproic acid, and carbamazepine, or second-generation antipsychotics.

KEY FACT

Side effects of lithium include:

- Weight gain
- Tremor
- Gastrointestinal disturbances
- Fatigue
- Cardiac arrhythmias
- Seizures
- Goiter/Hypothyroidism
- Leukocytosis (benign)
- Coma (in toxic doses)
- Polyuria (nephrogenic diabetes insipidus)
- Polydipsia
- Alopecia
- Metallic taste

Note: Lithium's toxidrome has a similar presentation though it is more severe.

WARDS TIP

The following mood stabilizers require monitoring of blood concentrations to guide dose adjustments. The therapeutic range is simple to remember with the 8 and 12 rule:

Lithium: 0.8–1.2 mEq/L
Carbamazapine: 8–12 mcg/mL
Valproic acid: 80–120 mcg/mL

KEY FACT

ECT is the best treatment for a pregnant woman who is having a manic episode. It provides a good alternative to antipsychotics and can be used with relative safety in all trimesters.

KEY FACT

A patient with a history of postpartum mania has a high risk of relapse with future deliveries and should be treated with mood stabilizing agents as prophylaxis. However, some of these medications may be contraindicated in breastfeeding.

KEY FACT

Rapid cycling is defined by the occurrence of four or more mood episodes (major depressive, hypomanic, or manic) in 1 year.

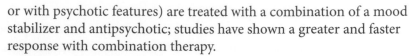

or with psychotic features) are treated with a combination of a mood stabilizer and antipsychotic; studies have shown a greater and faster response with combination therapy.

- Antidepressants are discouraged as monotherapy due to concerns of activating mania or hypomania. They are occasionally used to treat depressive episodes when patients concurrently take mood stabilizers.
- **Psychotherapy:** Supportive psychotherapy, family therapy, group therapy (may prolong remission once the acute manic episode has been controlled).
- **ECT:**
  - Works quickly in treatment of manic episodes.
  - Some patients require more treatments (up to 20) than for depression.
  - Especially effective for refractory or life-threatening acute mania or depression.
  - Like lithium, ECT reduces suicide risk.

BIPOLAR II DISORDER

Alternatively thought of as **recurrent MDEs with hypomania.**

Diagnosis and DSM-5 Criteria

History of one or more MDEs and at least one **hypomanic** episode. *Remember:* If there has been a full manic episode, *even in the past,* or if the patient ever has a history of psychosis, then the diagnosis is bipolar I, *not* bipolar II disorder.

Epidemiology

- Prevalence is unclear, with some studies showing greater and others less prevalence than bipolar I.
- May be slightly more common in women.
- Onset usually before age 30.
- No ethnic differences seen.
- Frequently misdiagnosed as unipolar depression and thereby inappropriately treated.

Etiology

Same as bipolar I disorder (see above).

Course and Prognosis

Tends to be chronic, requiring long-term treatment. Likely better prognosis than bipolar I given the lack of overt manic episodes.

Treatment

Fewer studies focus on the treatment for bipolar II. Currently, treatment is the same as bipolar I disorder (see above).

SPECIFIERS FOR BIPOLAR DISORDERS

- **Anxious distress:** Defined by feeling keyed up/tense, restless, difficulty concentrating, fears of something bad happening, and feelings of loss of control.
- **Mixed features:** Depressive symptoms present during the majority of days during mania/hypomania: dysphoria/depressed mood, anhedonia,

psychomotor retardation, fatigue/loss of energy, feelings of worthlessness or inappropriate guilt, thoughts of death or suicidal ideation.

- **Rapid cycling:** At least four mood episodes (manic, hypomanic, depressed) within 12 months.
- **Melancholic features** *(during depressed episode)*: Characterized by *anhedonia*, early morning awakenings, depression worse in the morning, psychomotor disturbance, excessive guilt, and anorexia.
- **Atypical features** *(during depressed episode)*: Characterized by hypersomnia, hyperphagia, reactive mood, leaden paralysis, and hypersensitivity to interpersonal rejection.
- **Psychotic features:** Characterized by the presence of delusions and/or hallucinations.
- **Catatonia:** Catalepsy, purposeless motor activity, extreme negativism or mutism, bizarre postures, and echolalia. Especially responsive to ECT.
- **Peripartum onset:** Onset of manic or hypomanic symptoms occurs during pregnancy or 4 weeks following delivery.
- **Seasonal pattern:** Temporal relationship between onset of mania/ hypomania and particular time of the year.

PERSISTENT DEPRESSIVE DISORDER (DYSTHYMIA)

Patients with persistent depressive disorder (dysthymia) have chronic depression most of the time, and they may have discrete MDEs.

Diagnosis and DSM-5 Criteria

1. Depressed mood for the majority of time most days for at least 2 years (in children or adolescents for at least 1 year).
2. At least two of the following:
   - Poor concentration or difficulty making decisions.
   - Feelings of hopelessness.
   - Poor appetite or overeating.
   - Insomnia or hypersomnia.
   - Low energy or fatigue.
   - Low self-esteem.
3. During the 2-year period:
   - The person has not been without the above symptoms for >2 months at a time.
   - May have MDE(s) or meet criteria for major depression continuously.
   - The patient must never have had a manic or hypomanic episode (this would make the diagnosis bipolar disorder or cyclothymic disorder, respectively).

Epidemiology

- Twelve-month prevalence: 2%.
- More common in women.
- Onset often in childhood, adolescence, and early adulthood.

Course and Prognosis

Early and insidious onset, with a chronic course. Depressive symptoms much less likely to resolve than in MDD.

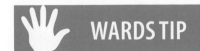 **WARDS TIP**

Bipolar I disorder may have psychotic features (delusions or hallucinations); these can occur during major depressive *or* manic episodes, but not in between. Remember to always include bipolar disorder in the differential diagnoses of a psychotic patient.

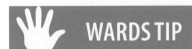 **WARDS TIP**

Schizoaffective disorder is characterized by psychosis with mood symptoms that are **only** present during *psychotic* episodes, while major depression with psychotic features is characterized by depression with psychosis **only** during *depressive* episodes. Remember this by looking at the word order: **schizo**affective is **psychosis** as the main symptom, and **depression** with psychotic features has **depression** as the main symptom.

WARDS TIP

Persistent *D*epressive *D*isorder (*DD*) = 2 *D*s
2 years of depression
2 listed criteria
Never asymptomatic for >2 months

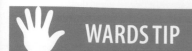

WARDS TIP

Symptoms of persistent depressive disorder (dysthymia)—two or more of:
CHASES
Poor **C**oncentration or difficulty making decisions
Feelings of **H**opelessness
Poor **A**ppetite or overeating
In**S**omnia or hypersomnia
Low **E**nergy or fatigue
Low **S**elf-esteem

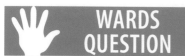

WARDS QUESTION

Q: What is the difference between bipolar I and bipolar II disorder?
A: Bipolar I disorder requires at least one *manic* episode but not necessarily a MDE, whereas bipolar II disorder requires both a *hypo*manic episode plus at least one *MDE*.

Treatment

- Combination treatment with psychotherapy and pharmacotherapy is more efficacious than either alone.
- Cognitive therapy, interpersonal therapy, and insight-oriented psychotherapy are the most effective.
- Antidepressants found to be beneficial include SSRIs, SNRIs, novel antidepressants (e.g., bupropion, mirtazapine), TCAs, and MAOIs.

CYCLOTHYMIC DISORDER

Alternating periods of hypomania and periods with mild-to-moderate depressive symptoms.

Diagnosis and DSM-5 Criteria

- Numerous periods with hypomanic symptoms (but not a full hypomanic episode) and periods with depressive symptoms (but not full MDE) for at least 2 years.
- The person must never have been symptom free for >2 months during those 2 years.
- No history of MDE, hypomania, or manic episode.

Epidemiology

- Lifetime prevalence: <1%.
- May coexist with borderline personality disorder.
- Onset usually between ages 15 and 25.
- Occurs equally in males and females.

Course and Prognosis
Chronic course; approximately one-third of patients eventually develop bipolar I/II disorder.

Treatment
Antimanic agents (mood stabilizers or second-generation antipsychotics) are used to treat bipolar disorder (see above).

PREMENSTRUAL DYSPHORIC DISORDER

Mood lability, irritability, dysphoria, and anxiety that occur repeatedly during the premenstrual phase of the cycle.

Diagnosis and DSM-5 Criteria

- In most menstrual cycles, at least five symptoms (below) are present in the final week before menses, improve within a few days after menses, and are minimal/absent in the week postmenses (should be confirmed by daily ratings for at least two menstrual cycles).
- At least one of the following symptoms is present: affective lability, irritability/anger, depressed mood, anxiety/tension.
- At least one of the following symptoms is present (for total of at least five symptoms when combined with above): anhedonia, problems concentrating, anergia, appetite changes/food cravings, hypersomnia/insomnia, feeling overwhelmed/out of control, physical symptoms (e.g., breast tenderness/swelling, joint/muscle pain, bloating, weight gain).

- Symptoms cause clinically significant distress or impairment in functioning.
- Symptoms are not only exacerbation of another disorder (e.g., MDD, panic disorder, persistent depressive disorder).
- Symptoms are not due to a substance (medication or drug) or another medical condition.

Epidemiology/Etiology

- Prevalence: 1.8%.
- Onset can occur at any time after menarche.
- Has been observed worldwide.
- Environmental and genetic factors contribute.

Course and Prognosis

Symptoms may worsen prior to menopause but cease after menopause.

Treatment

SSRIs are first-line treatment, either as daily therapy or luteal phase-only treatment (starting on cycle day 14 and stopping upon menses or shortly thereafter). Oral contraceptives may reduce symptoms. Gonadotropin-releasing hormone (GnRH) agonists have also been used, and, in rare, severe cases, bilateral oophorectomy with hysterectomy will resolve symptoms.

DISRUPTIVE MOOD DYSREGULATION DISORDER (DMDD)

Chronic, severe, persistent irritability occurring in childhood and adolescence.

Diagnosis and DSM-5 Criteria

- Severe recurrent verbal and/or physical outbursts out of proportion to situation.
- Outbursts ≥3 per week and inconsistent with developmental level.
- Mood between outbursts is persistently angry/irritable most of the day nearly every day, and is observed by others.
- Symptoms for at least 1 year, and no more than 3 months without symptoms.
- Symptoms in at least two settings (e.g., home, school, peers).
- Symptoms must have started before age 10, but diagnosis can be made from ages 6 to 18.
- No episodes meeting full criteria for manic/hypomanic episode lasting longer than 1 day.
- Behaviors do not occur during MDD and not better explained by another mental disorder (this disorder cannot coexist with oppositional defiant disorder, intermittent explosive disorder, or bipolar disorder).
- Symptoms not due to a substance (medication or drug) or another medical condition.

Epidemiology/Etiology

- Prevalence is unclear as this is a newer diagnosis.
- 6–12-month prevalence rates of chronic/severe persistent irritability in children: 2–5%.
- Rates likely greater in males than females.

Course and Prognosis

- By definition, DMDD must occur prior to 10 years of age.
- Approximately 50% of those with DMDD continue to meet criteria after 1 year.
- Rates of conversion to bipolar disorder are very low.
- Very high rates of comorbidity, especially with ADHD, MDD, and substance use disorders.

Treatment

- Given the newer nature of this diagnosis, there are no consensus evidenced-based treatments. Psychotherapy (such as parent management training) for the patient and family is generally first line.
- Medications should be used to treat comorbid disorders.
- Stimulants, SSRIs, mood stabilizers, and second-generation antipsychotics have all been used to treat the primary symptoms of DMDD.

OTHER DISORDERS OF MOOD IN *DSM-5*

- Mood disorder due to another medical condition.
- Substance/Medication-induced mood disorder.
- Specified depressive/bipolar disorder (meets criteria for MDE or bipolar except shorter duration or too few symptoms)
- Unspecified depressive/bipolar disorder.

CHAPTER 5

ANXIETY, OBSESSIVE-COMPULSIVE, TRAUMA, AND
STRESSOR-RELATED DISORDERS

WARDS TIP

Assess for psychopathology if an individual's symptoms are causing **S**ocial and/or **O**ccupational **D**ysfunction (use mnemonic **SOD**).

WARDS TIP

Late-onset anxiety symptoms without a prior history or family psychiatric history should increase suspicion of anxiety caused by another medical condition or substance use.

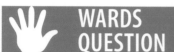

WARDS QUESTION

Q: In a patient with comorbid anxiety and depression, would treatment with a benzodiazepine be a first-line treatment?
A: No. Avoid use of benzodiazepines because they may worsen depression.

Anxiety Disorders

Anxiety disorders are characterized by excessive or inappropriate fear or anxiety. *Fear* is manifested by a transient increase in sympathetic activity ("fight or flight" physiologic response, thoughts, feelings, behaviors) in a situation perceived as dangerous or threatening. By contrast, *anxiety* involves apprehension regarding the possibility of a negative future event. The criteria for most anxiety disorders involve symptoms that cause **clinically significant distress** or **impairment in social and/or occupational functioning** (see Table 5-1). *DSM-5* anxiety disorders include generalized anxiety disorder, panic disorder, agoraphobia, social anxiety disorder, selective mutism, and specific phobias.

- Anxiety disorders are caused by a combination of genetic, biological, environmental, and psychosocial factors.

- Primary anxiety disorders are diagnosed after determining that symptoms are NOT due to the physiological effects of a substance, medication (see Table 5-2), or another medical condition (see Table 5-3).

- Major neurotransmitter systems implicated: norepinephrine (NE), serotonin (5-HT), and gamma-aminobutyric acid (GABA).

TABLE 5-1. Signs and Symptoms of Anxiety	
Constitutional	Fatigue, diaphoresis, shivering
Cardiac	Chest pain, palpitations, tachycardia, hypertension
Pulmonary	Shortness of breath, hyperventilation
Neurologic/ musculoskeletal	Vertigo, light-headedness, paresthesias, tremors, insomnia, muscle tension
Gastrointestinal	Abdominal discomfort, anorexia, nausea, emesis, diarrhea, constipation

TABLE 5-2. Medications and Substances That Cause Anxiety	
Alcohol	Intoxication/withdrawal
Sedatives, hypnotics, or anxiolytics	Withdrawal
Cannabis	Intoxication
Hallucinogens (PCP, LSD, MDMA)	Intoxication
Stimulants (amphetamines, cocaine)	Intoxication/withdrawal
Caffeine	Intoxication/withdrawal
Tobacco	Intoxication/withdrawal
Opioids	Withdrawal

LSD, lysergic acid diethylamide; MDMA, 3,4-methylenedioxy methamphetamine; PCP, phencyclidine.

TABLE 5-3. Medical Conditions That Cause Anxiety	
Neurologic	Epilepsy, migraines, brain tumors, multiple sclerosis, Huntington disease
Endocrine	Hyperthyroidism, hypoglycemia, pheochromocytoma, carcinoid syndrome
Metabolic	Vitamin B12 deficiency, electrolyte abnormalities, porphyria
Respiratory	Asthma, chronic obstructive pulmonary disease (COPD), hypoxia, pulmonary embolism (PE), pneumonia, pneumothorax
Cardiovascular	Congestive heart failure (CHF), angina, arrhythmia, myocardial infarction (MI)

- Most common form of psychopathology.
- More frequently seen in women compared to men, approximately 2:1 ratio.

Treatment Guidelines

- Determine treatment course based on the severity of symptoms.
- Initiate psychotherapy for mild anxiety.
- Consider a **combination** of therapy and medication **for moderate to severe anxiety**.

Pharmacotherapy

- **Selective serotonin reuptake inhibitors (SSRIs)** (e.g., sertraline) and **serotonin-norepinephrine reuptake inhibitors (SNRIs)** (e.g., venlafaxine) are **first-line** medications.
- **Benzodiazepines** can be used as an adjunctive short-term treatment to achieve acute reduction of severe anxiety symptoms (e.g., while getting stabilized on an SSRI), but regular use can result in dependence. Therefore, minimize the use, duration, and dose, and avoid in patients with a history of substance use disorders, particularly alcohol.
- Mechanism of action: Enhance activity of GABA at GABA-A receptor.
- In patients with comorbid substance use consider nonaddictive anxiolytic alternatives for PRN use, such as gabapentin and antihistamines with anxiolytic properties (e.g., diphenhydramine or hydroxyzine).
- **Buspirone** is a non-benzodiazepine anxiolytic which has partial agonist activity at the 5-HT$_{1A}$ receptor. Due to minimal efficacy as monotherapy, buspirone is typically prescribed only as augmentation.
- **Beta-blockers (e.g., propranolol)** may be used to help control autonomic symptoms (e.g., palpitations, tachycardia, sweating) of **panic attacks** or **performance anxiety**.
- **Tricyclic antidepressants** (TCAs) and **monoamine oxidase inhibitors** (MAOIs) may be considered if first-line agents are not effective. Their side-effect profile, especially cardiovascular effects, makes them less tolerable and more dangerous.

Psychotherapy

- Many modalities of psychotherapy are helpful for patients suffering from anxiety disorders.
  - **Cognitive-behavioral therapy (CBT)** has proven effective for anxiety disorders. CBT examines the relationship between anxiety-driven cognitions (thoughts), emotions, and behavior.
  - **Psychodynamic psychotherapy** facilitates insight into the development of anxiety symptoms, leading to more adaptive coping styles and subsequent improvement over time.

PANIC ATTACKS

A panic attack is a fear response involving a sudden onset of intense anxiety which may either be triggered or occur spontaneously. Panic attacks peak

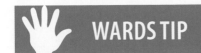

WARDS TIP

Use *benzodiazepines* to temporarily *bridge* patients until long-term medication becomes effective.

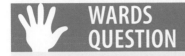

WARDS QUESTION

Q: How long does it take for SSRIs to typically become fully effective? **A:** About 4–6 weeks.

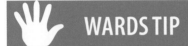

WARDS TIP

The goal of medication treatment is to achieve symptomatic relief and continue treatment for at least 6 months before attempting to titrate off medications.

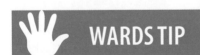

WARDS TIP

Medications can reduce symptoms sufficiently so that a patient can participate and learn the skills offered in therapy. Therapy can additionally be used as maintenance treatment to prevent relapse.

KEY FACT

**Symptoms of panic attacks
Da PANICS**

Dizziness, **d**isconnectedness, **d**erealization (unreality), **d**epersonalization (detached from self)

Palpitations, **p**aresthesias

Abdominal distress

Numbness, **n**ausea

Intense fear of dying, losing control or "going crazy"

Chills, **c**hest pain

Sweating, **s**haking, **s**hortness of breath

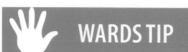

WARDS TIP

Use the *Bs* to *Block* the *Ps*: *Beta-Blockers* for *Panic* attacks and *Performance* anxiety.

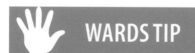

WARDS TIP

Smoking is a risk factor for panic attacks.

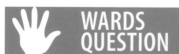

WARDS QUESTION

Q: When a patient presents with the new onset of a panic attack, what potentially life-threatening medical conditions should be ruled out?
A: Heart attack, cardiac arrhythmia, electrolyte dysfunction, hypoglycemia, thyrotoxicosis, and pulmonary embolism.

within minutes and usually resolve within half an hour. Patients may continue to feel anxious for hours afterwards and believe they are experiencing a prolonged panic attack. Although classically associated with panic disorder, panic attacks can also be experienced with other psychiatric disorders and medical conditions.

PANIC DISORDER

Panic disorder is diagnosed in patients who experience *spontaneous*, recurrent panic attacks and who are fearful of reoccurring attacks. These attacks most often occur suddenly, *out of the blue*, although they may sometimes have a clear trigger. The frequency of attacks ranges from multiple times per day to a few times per month. The keystone feature of panic disorder is that patients develop debilitating anticipatory anxiety about having future attacks—"fear of the fear."

Diagnosis and DSM-5 Criteria

- **Recurrent, *unexpected* panic attacks** without an identifiable trigger.
- One or more of panic attacks followed by ≥1 month of continuous worry about experiencing subsequent attacks or their consequences, and/or a maladaptive change in behaviors (e.g., avoidance of possible triggers).
- Not due to the physiological effects of a substance, another medical or neurological condition (e.g., traumatic brain injury), or another mental disorder.

Etiology

- Genetic factors: Greater risk of panic disorder if a first-degree relative is affected.
- Psychosocial factors: Increased incidence of stressors (especially loss) prior to onset of disorder; history of childhood physical or sexual abuse.

Epidemiology

- Lifetime prevalence: 4%.
- Higher rates in woman compared to men, approximately 2:1.
- Median age of onset: 20–24 years old.

Course and Prognosis

- Panic disorder has a chronic course with waxing and waning symptoms.
- Relapses are common with discontinuation of medication.
- Only a minority of patients have full remission of symptoms.
- Up to 65% of patients with panic disorder also have major depression.
- Additional comorbid syndromes include other anxiety disorders (e.g., agoraphobia), bipolar disorder, and alcohol use disorder.

Treatment

Combination of CBT and Pharmacotherapy = most effective.

- First-line: **SSRIs** (e.g., sertraline, citalopram, escitalopram).
- **SNRIs** (e.g., venlafaxine, desvenlafaxine, duloxetine) are also efficacious.
- If the above options are not effective, can consider TCAs (e.g., clomipramine, imipramine).
- Can use benzodiazepines (e.g., clonazepam, lorazepam) as scheduled or PRN, until other medications reach therapeutic efficacy.

AGORAPHOBIA

Agoraphobia is an intense fear of being in public places where escape or obtaining help may be difficult. It often develops with panic disorder. The course of the disorder is usually chronic. Avoidance behaviors may become as extreme as complete confinement to the home.

Diagnosis and DSM-5 Criteria

- Intense fear/anxiety about at least two situations due to concerns of difficulty escaping or obtaining help in case of panic or other humiliating symptoms:
  - Outside of the home alone.
  - Open spaces (e.g., bridges).
  - Enclosed places (e.g., stores).
  - Public transportation (e.g., trains).
  - Crowds/lines.
- The triggering situations cause fear/anxiety that is out of proportion to the potential danger posed, leading to endurance of intense anxiety, avoidance, or need for a companion. This holds true even if the patient suffers from another medical condition such as inflammatory bowel disease (IBS), which may lead to embarrassing public scenarios.
- Symptoms cause significant social or occupational dysfunction.
- Symptoms last ≥6 months.
- Symptoms not better explained by another mental disorder.

Etiology

- Strong genetic factor: Heritability about 60%.
- Psychosocial factor: Onset frequently follows a traumatic event.

Course/Prognosis

- More than 50% of patients experience a panic attack prior to developing agoraphobia.
- Onset is usually before age 35.
- Course is persistent and chronic, with rare full remission.
- Comorbid diagnoses include other anxiety disorders, depressive disorders, and substance use disorders.

Treatment

- CBT and SSRIs

SPECIFIC PHOBIAS

A phobia is defined as an **irrational fear that leads to endurance of the anxiety and/or avoidance** of the feared object or situation. A *specific phobia* is an intense fear of a specific object or situation (i.e., the phobic stimulus).

Diagnosis and DSM-5 Criteria

- Persistent, excessive fear elicited by a specific situation or object which is out of proportion to any actual danger/threat.
- Exposure to the situation triggers an immediate fear response.
- Situation or object is avoided when possible or tolerated with intense anxiety.

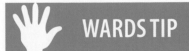

WARDS TIP

A classic panic disorder case involves a woman who repeatedly visits the ER because she is afraid of dying when she experiences episodes of palpitations, diaphoresis, and shortness of breath. The patient has no prior medical history and the medical workup is negative.

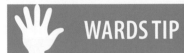

WARDS TIP

Carefully screen patients with panic attacks for suicidality. They are at an increased risk for suicide attempts.

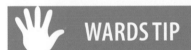

WARDS TIP

Start SSRIs or SNRIs at low doses and ↑ slowly because side effects may initially worsen anxiety, especially in panic disorder.

KEY FACT

Characteristic situations avoided in agoraphobia include bridges, crowds, buses, trains, or any open areas outside the home.

KEY FACT

Common Domains of Social Anxiety Disorder (Social Phobia):

- Speaking in public.
- Eating in public.
- Using public restrooms.

KEY FACT

Common Specific Phobias:
Animal—spiders, insects, dogs, snakes, and mice.
Natural environment—heights, storms, and water.
Situational—elevators, airplanes, buses, and enclosed spaces.
Blood-injection-injury—needles, injections, blood, injuries, and invasive medical procedures.

WARDS TIP

Patients with blood-injury- injection-specific phobia (fear of needles, etc.) may experience bradycardia and hypotension leading to vasovagal syncope.

KEY FACT

Substance use and depressive disorders frequently co-occur with phobias.

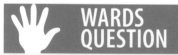

WARDS QUESTION

Q: What medication often successfully treats performance anxiety?
A: Beta-blockers.

- Symptoms cause significant social or occupational dysfunction.
- Duration ≥6 months.
- Not due to the physiological effects of a substance, another medical or neurological condition (e.g., traumatic brain injury), or another mental disorder.

Epidemiology

- Phobias are the **most common psychiatric disorder** in women and second most common in men (substance-related is first).
- Lifetime prevalence of specific phobia: >10%.
- Mean age of onset for specific phobia is 10 years.
- Specific phobia rates are higher in women compared to men (2:1) but vary depending on the type of stimulus.

Treatment

- Treatment of choice: CBT with exposure.

SOCIAL ANXIETY DISORDER (SOCIAL PHOBIA)

Social anxiety disorder (social phobia) is the **fear of scrutiny by others or fear of acting in a humiliating or embarrassing way**. The phobia may develop in the wake of negative or traumatic encounters with the stimulus. Social situations causing significant anxiety may be avoided altogether, resulting in social and academic/occupational impairment.

The diagnostic criteria for **social anxiety disorder (social phobia)** are similar to specific phobia except the phobic stimulus is related to *social scrutiny and negative evaluation*. The patients fear embarrassment, humiliation, and rejection. This fear may be limited to performance or public speaking, which may be routinely encountered in the patient's occupation or academic pursuit.

Epidemiology

- Median age of onset for social anxiety disorder is 13 years.
- Social anxiety disorder occurs equally across genders.

Treatment

- Treatment of choice: CBT.
- First-line medication, if needed: SSRIs (e.g., sertraline, fluoxetine) or SNRIs (e.g., venlafaxine) for debilitating symptoms.
- Benzodiazepines (e.g., clonazepam, lorazepam) can be used as scheduled or PRN.
- Beta-blockers (e.g., atenolol, propranolol) PRN for performance anxiety/ public speaking.

SELECTIVE MUTISM

Selective mutism is a rare condition characterized by a failure to speak in specific situations for at least 1 month, despite the intact ability to comprehend and use language. Symptom onset typically starts during childhood. The majority of these patients suffer from anxiety, particularly social anxiety, as the mutism manifests in social settings. The patients may remain completely silent or just whisper. They may use nonverbal means of communication, such as writing or gesturing.

Diagnosis and DSM-5 Criteria

- Consistent failure to speak in select social situations (e.g., school) despite speech ability in other scenarios.
- Mutism is not due to a language difficulty or a communication disorder.
- Symptoms cause significant impairment in academic, occupational, or social functioning.
- Symptoms last >1 month (extending beyond first month of school).

Treatment

- Psychotherapy: CBT, family therapy.
- Medications: SSRIs (especially with comorbid social anxiety disorder).

SEPARATION ANXIETY DISORDER

As part of normal human development, infants become distressed when they are separated from their primary caregiver. *Stranger anxiety* begins around 6 months and peaks around 9 months, while *separation anxiety* typically emerges by 1 year of age and peaks by 18 months. However, when the anxiety due to separation becomes extreme or developmentally inappropriate, it is considered pathologic. Separation anxiety disorder may be preceded by a stressful life event.

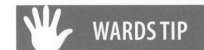

WARDS TIP

Separation anxiety may lead to complaints of somatic symptoms to avoid school/work.

Diagnosis and DSM-5 Criteria

Excessive and developmentally inappropriate fear/anxiety regarding **separation from attachment figures**, with at least three of the following:

- Separation from attachment figures leads to extreme distress.
- Excessive worry about loss of or harm to attachment figures.
- Excessive worry about experiencing an event that leads to separation from attachment figures.
- Reluctance to leave home or attend school or work.
- Reluctance to be alone.
- Reluctance to sleep alone or away from home.
- Complaints of physical symptoms when separated from major attachment figures.
- Nightmares of separation and refusal to sleep without proximity to attachment figure.
- Lasts for ≥4 weeks in children/adolescents and ≥6 months in adults.
- Symptoms cause significant social, academic, or occupational dysfunction.
- Symptoms not due to another mental disorder.

Treatment

- Psychotherapy: CBT, family therapy.
- Medications: SSRIs can be effective as an adjunct to therapy.

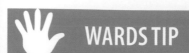

WARDS TIP

GAD Mnemonic
Worry WARTS
Wound up, **w**orn-out
Absent-minded
Restless
Tense
Sleepless

A 24-year-old law student presents to an outpatient psychiatry clinic with a chief complaint that she is "so stressed out, worrying about everything." She is overwhelmed with her academic workload and upcoming exams. She has had trouble falling asleep and feels chronically fatigued. The patient also suffers from frequent headaches and muscle tightness in her neck and shoulders.

The patient's husband describes her as "a worrier. She's always concerned about me getting into an accident, her flunking out of school, not finding a job—the list goes on."

The patient reports that she has always had some degree of anxiety, but previously found it motivating. Over the last year since law school began, her symptoms have become debilitating.

What is the most likely diagnosis?

With the patient's history of *excessive worrying* about *everything,* the most likely diagnosis is generalized anxiety disorder (GAD). Like many patients with GAD, she is described as a *worrier.* She reports typical associated symptoms: insomnia, fatigue, and impaired concentration. Her symptoms have been present for over *6 months.*

What is the next step?

A complete physical exam and medical workup should be performed to rule out other medical conditions or substance use contributing to or causing her anxiety symptoms.

What are treatment options?

Treatment options for GAD include psychotherapy (usually CBT) and pharmacotherapy (typically SSRIs). A combination of both modalities may achieve better remission rates than either treatment alone.

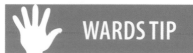

WARDS TIP

For patients with anxiety, evaluate for caffeine use and recommend significant reduction or elimination.

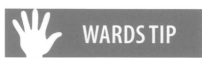

WARDS TIP

Exercise can significantly reduce anxiety.

WARDS TIP

The worries associated with *GAD* are free-floating across various areas, as opposed to being fixed on a specific trigger.

GENERALIZED ANXIETY DISORDER (GAD)

Patients with GAD have persistent, excessive anxiety about many aspects of their daily lives. Commonly associated physical symptoms include fatigue and muscle tension, which often lead to an initial presentation to primary care.

Diagnosis and DSM-5 Criteria

- Excessive anxiety/worry about various daily events/activities ≥6 months.
- Difficulty controlling worry.
- Associated ≥3 symptoms: restlessness, fatigue, impaired concentration, irritability, muscle tension, insomnia.
- Not due to the physiological effects of a substance, another medical or neurological condition (e.g., traumatic brain injury), or another mental disorder.
- Symptoms cause significant social or occupational dysfunction.

Epidemiology/Etiology

- Lifetime prevalence: 5–9%.
- GAD rates higher in women compared to men (2:1).
- One-third of risk for developing GAD is genetic.

Course/Prognosis

- Symptoms of worry begin in childhood.
- Median age of onset of GAD: 30 years.
- Course is chronic, with waxing and waning symptoms.
- Rates of full remission are low.
- GAD is highly comorbid with other anxiety and depressive disorders.

Treatment

The most effective treatment approach combines psychotherapy and pharmacotherapy:

- CBT.
- SSRIs (e.g., sertraline, citalopram) or SNRIs (e.g., venlafaxine, duloxetine).
- Can also consider a short-term course of benzodiazepines or augmentation with buspirone.
- Much less commonly used medications are TCAs and MAOIs.

Obsessive-Compulsive and Related Disorders

OBSESSIVE-COMPULSIVE DISORDER (OCD)

OCD is characterized by obsessions and/or compulsions that are time-consuming, distressing, and impairing. **Obsessions** are recurrent, intrusive, and undesired thoughts that increase anxiety. Patients may attempt to relieve the anxiety by performing **compulsions**, which are repetitive behaviors or mental rituals. Anxiety may increase when a patient resists acting out a compulsion. Patients with OCD have varying degrees of insight.

Diagnosis and DSM-5 Criteria

- Experiencing obsessions and/or compulsions that are time-consuming (e.g., >1 hr/day) and cause significant distress or dysfunction.
  - **Obsessions:** Recurrent, intrusive, anxiety-provoking thoughts, images, or urges that the patient attempts to suppress, ignore, or neutralize by some other thought or action (i.e., by performing a compulsion).
  - **Compulsions:** Repetitive behaviors or mental acts the patient feels driven to perform in response to an obsession, or a rule aimed at stress reduction or disaster prevention. The behaviors are excessive and/or not realistically connected to what they are meant to prevent.
- Not due to the physiological effects of a substance, another medical or neurological condition (e.g., traumatic brain injury), or another mental disorder.

Epidemiology

- Lifetime prevalence: 2–3%.
- No gender difference in prevalence overall.

Etiology

- Significant genetic component: Higher rates of OCD in first-degree relatives and monozygotic twins than in the general population. Higher rate of OCD in first-degree relatives with Tourette's disorder.

Course/Prognosis

- Chronic, with waxing and waning symptoms.
- Less than 20% remission rate without treatment.
- Suicidal ideation in 50% and suicide attempts in 25% of patients with OCD.
- High comorbidity with other anxiety disorders, depressive or bipolar disorder, obsessive-compulsive personality disorder, and tic disorder.

Treatment

Utilize a combination of psychopharmacology and CBT.

KEY FACT

Compulsions can often take the form of repeated checking or counting.

KEY FACT

Patients with OCD often initially seek help from primary care and other nonpsychiatric providers for help with the consequences of compulsions (e.g., excessive washing).

KEY FACT

The triad of "uncontrollable urges"—OCD, ADHD, and tic disorder—are usually first seen in children or adolescents.

KEY FACTS

Common Patterns of Obsessions and Compulsions

Obsessions	Compulsions
Contamination	Cleaning or avoidance of contaminant
Doubt or harm	Checking multiple times to avoid potential danger
Symmetry	Ordering or counting
Intrusive, taboo thoughts	With or without related compulsion

KEY FACT

Differentiating OCD and obsessive-compulsive personality disorder (OCPD):
- Individuals with OCPD are obsessed with details, control, and perfectionism without experiencing unwanted preoccupations or compulsions.
- OCD patients are *dis*tressed by their symptoms (ego-*dys*tonic).

CBT focuses on *exposure and response prevention*: prolonged, graded exposure to ritual-eliciting stimulus and prevention of the relieving compulsion.

- First-line medication: SSRIs (e.g., sertraline, fluoxetine), typically at higher doses.
- Second-line agents: SNRIs (e.g., venlafaxine) or the most serotonin selective **TCA, clomipramine.**
- Can augment with atypical antipsychotics in severe cases.
- In debilitating, treatment-resistant cases, consider psychosurgery (cingulotomy) or electroconvulsive therapy (ECT).

BODY DYSMORPHIC DISORDER

- Patients with body dysmorphic disorder are preoccupied with nonexistent or minor physical defects that they regard as severe, grotesque, and repulsive.
- These individuals spend significant time trying to correct perceived flaws with makeup, dermatological procedures, or plastic surgery.

Diagnosis and DSM-5 Criteria

- Preoccupation with one or more perceived defects or flaws in physical appearance that are not observable by or appear slight to others.
- In response to the appearance concerns, repetitive behaviors (e.g., skin picking, excessive grooming) or mental acts (e.g., comparing appearance to others) are performed.
- Preoccupation causes significant distress or impairment in functioning.
- Appearance preoccupation is not better accounted for by concerns with body fat/weight in an eating disorder.

Epidemiology

- Slightly more common in women than men.
- Prevalence elevated in those with high rates of childhood abuse and neglect.
- Increased risk in first-degree relatives of patients with OCD.
- Higher prevalence in dermatologic and cosmetic surgery patients.
- Mean age of onset: 15 years.

Course/Prognosis

- The onset is usually gradual, beginning in early adolescence. Symptoms tend to be chronic.
- Surgical or dermatological procedures are routinely unsuccessful in satisfying the patient.
- High rate of suicidal ideation and attempts.
- Comorbidity with major depression, social anxiety disorder (social phobia), and OCD.

Treatment

- SSRIs and/or CBT may reduce the obsessive and compulsive symptoms in many patients.

HOARDING DISORDER

Diagnosis and DSM-5 Criteria

- Persistent difficulty discarding possessions, regardless of value.
- Difficulty is due to need to save the items and distress associated with discarding them.

- Results in accumulation of possessions that congest/clutter living areas and compromise use.
- Hoarding causes clinically significant distress or impairment in social, occupational, or other areas of functioning.
- Hoarding is not attributable to another medical condition or another mental disorder.

Epidemiology/Etiology

- Point prevalence of significant hoarding is 2–6%.
- Hoarding is three times more prevalent in the elderly population.
- Onset often preceded by stressful and traumatic events.
- **50%** of individuals with hoarding have at least one hoarding relative.

Course/Prognosis

- Hoarding behavior begins in early teens and tends to worsen over time.
- Usually chronic course.
- 75% of individuals have comorbid mood (MDD) or anxiety disorder (social anxiety disorder).
- 20% of individuals have comorbid OCD.

Treatment

- Very difficult to treat.
- Specialized CBT for hoarding.
- SSRIs can be used.

TRICHOTILLOMANIA (HAIR-PULLING DISORDER)

Diagnosis and DSM-5 Criteria

- Recurrent pulling out of one's hair, resulting in hair loss.
- Repeated attempts to decrease or stop hair pulling.
- Causes significant distress or impairment in daily functioning.
- Hair pulling or hair loss is not due to another medical condition or psychiatric disorder.
- Usually involves the scalp, eyebrows, or eyelashes. May include facial, axillary, or pubic hair.

Epidemiology/Etiology

- Lifetime prevalence: 1–2% of the adult population.
- More common in women than in men (10:1 ratio).
- Onset usually at puberty and frequently associated with a stressful event.
- Etiology may involve biological, genetic, and environmental factors.
- Increased incidence of comorbid OCD, major depressive disorder, and excoriation (skin-picking) disorder.
- Course may be chronic with waxing and waning periods. Adult onset is generally more difficult to treat.

Treatment

- **Recommended:** Specialized types of cognitive-behavior therapy (e.g., habit reversal training).
- Pharmacologic treatment includes SSRIs, second-generation antipsychotics, lithium, or *N*-acetylcysteine (NAC).

EXCORIATION (SKIN-PICKING) DISORDER

Diagnosis and DSM-5 Criteria

- Recurrent skin picking resulting in lesions.
- Repeated attempts to decrease or stop skin picking.
- Causes significant distress or impairment in daily functioning.
- Not due to the physiological effects of a substance, another medical or neurological condition (e.g., traumatic brain injury), or another mental disorder.

Epidemiology/Etiology

- Lifetime prevalence: 1.4% of the adult population.
- More than 75% of cases are women.
- More common in individuals with OCD and first-degree family members.

Course/Prognosis

- Skin picking begins in adolescence.
- Course is chronic with waxing and waning periods if untreated.
- Comorbidity with OCD, trichotillomania, and MDD.

Treatment

- Specialized types of cognitive-behavior therapy (e.g., habit reversal training).
- SSRIs have shown some benefit.

Trauma and Stressor-Related Disorders

 A 19-year-old freshman is brought to the ER by her college roommate due to her concerns that she "really needs to get some help—she hasn't been herself since a party we went to together." The freshman has been hyper-vigilant, tearful, and crying out so loudly in her sleep that she wakes up her peers. The roommate discloses concern that a traumatic incident occurred at a party last month. The patient is guarded and reluctant to talk about details. She reports that since the party, she has experienced intrusive thoughts and nightmares. The patient is afraid to leave her room, and feels on edge most of the time.

What is the most likely diagnosis?

The patient has been suffering from symptoms of posttraumatic stress disorder (PTSD) for the last month after a traumatic incident with associated low mood, avoidance, hypervigilance, intrusive thoughts, and nightmares.

POSTTRAUMATIC STRESS DISORDER (PTSD) AND ACUTE STRESS DISORDER

PTSD is characterized by the development of multiple symptoms after exposure to one or more traumatic events: intrusive symptoms (e.g., nightmares, flash-backs), avoidance, negative alterations in thoughts and mood, and increased arousal. The symptoms last for at least a month and may occur immediately after the trauma or with delayed expression.

Acute stress disorder is diagnosed in patients who experience a major trau-matic event and suffer from similar symptoms as PTSD (see Table 5-4) but for a shorter duration. The onset of symptoms occurs within 1 month of the trauma and **symptoms last for less than 1 month**.

TABLE 5-4. Posttraumatic Stress Disorder and Acute Stress Disorder	
Posttraumatic Stress Disorder	**Acute Stress Disorder**
Trauma occurred at any time in past	Trauma occurred <1 month ago
Symptoms last >1 month	Symptoms last <1 month

Diagnosis and DSM-5 Criteria

- Exposure to actual or threatened death, serious injury, or sexual violence by **directly experiencing or witnessing the trauma.**
- Recurrent intrusions of reexperiencing the event via memories, nightmares, or dissociative reactions (e.g., flashbacks); intense distress at exposure to cues relating to the trauma; or physiological reactions to cues relating to the trauma.
- Active avoidance of triggering stimuli (e.g., memories, feelings, people, places, objects) associated with the trauma.
- At least two of the following negative cognitions/mood: dissociative amnesia, negative feelings of self/others/world, self-blame, negative emotions (e.g., fear, horror, anger, guilt), anhedonia, feelings of detachment/estrangement, inability to experience positive emotions.
- At least two of the following symptoms of increased arousal/reactivity: hypervigilance, exaggerated startle response, irritability, angry outbursts, impaired concentration, insomnia.
- Symptoms not caused by the direct effects of a substance or another medical condition.
- Symptoms result in significant impairment in social or occupational functioning.
- The presentation differs in children <7 years of age.

Epidemiology/Etiology

- Lifetime prevalence of PTSD: >8%.
- Higher prevalence in women, most likely due to greater risk of exposure to traumatic events, particularly rape and other forms of interpersonal violence.
- Exposure to prior trauma, especially during childhood, is a risk factor for developing PTSD.

Course/Prognosis

- PTSD usually begins within 3 months after the trauma.
- Symptoms may manifest after a delayed expression.
- Fifty percent of patients with PTSD have complete recovery within 3 months.
- Symptoms tend to diminish with older age.
- Eighty percent of patients with PTSD have a comorbid mental disorder (e.g., MDD, bipolar disorder, anxiety disorder, substance use disorder).

Treatment

- **Pharmacological**
  - First-line antidepressants: SSRIs (e.g., sertraline) or SNRIs (e.g., venlafaxine).
  - Prazosin, α_1-receptor antagonist, targets nightmares and hypervigilance.
  - Consider augmentation with a second-generation antipsychotic in severe or treatment-resistant cases.

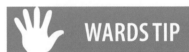

Q: What medication has shown some efficacy as an adjunct treatment for nightmares in patients with PTSD?
A: Prazosin.

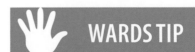

Criteria of PTSD: TRAUMA
Traumatic event
Reexperience
Avoidance
Unable to function
Month or more of symptoms
Arousal increased

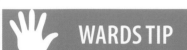

WARDS TIP

Cognitive processing therapy is a modified form of CBT in which thoughts, feelings, and meanings of the event are revisited and questioned.

WARDS TIP

Addictive medications such as benzodiazepines should be avoided in the treatment of PTSD because of the high rate of comorbid substance use disorders and the lack of efficacy.

KEY FACT

PTSD stressor = life threatening.

Adjustment disorder stressor ≠ life threatening.

■ **Psychotherapy**
- Specialized forms of CBT (e.g., exposure therapy, cognitive processing therapy).
- Supportive and psychodynamic therapy.
- Couples/family therapy.

ADJUSTMENT DISORDERS

Adjustment disorders occur when behavioral or emotional symptoms develop after a non-life-threatening, stressful life event (e.g., divorce, death of a loved one, or loss of a job).

Diagnosis and DSM-5 Criteria
1. Development of emotional or behavioral symptoms within 3 months in response to an identifiable stressful life event. These symptoms produce either:
   - Excessive distress in relation to the event.
   - Significant impairment in daily functioning.
2. The symptoms are not those of normal bereavement.
3. Symptoms resolve within 6 months after the stressor has terminated.
4. The stress-related disturbance does not meet criteria for another mental disorder.

Subtypes: Based on a predominance of either depressed mood, anxiety, mixed anxiety and depression, disturbance of conduct (such as aggression), or mixed disturbance of emotions and conduct.

Epidemiology
- 5–20% of patients in outpatient mental health clinics have an adjustment disorder.
- May occur at any age.

Etiology
- Triggered by psychosocial factors.

Prognosis
May be chronic if the stressor is chronic or recurrent.

Treatment
- Supportive psychotherapy.
- Group therapy.
- If clinically indicated, pharmacotherapy can target associated impairing symptoms (insomnia, anxiety, or depression).

WARDS TIP

Many people have odd tendencies and quirks. These are not pathological unless they cause significant distress or impairment in daily functioning.

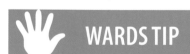

KEY FACT

Ego-syntonic refers to feelings, thoughts, and/or behaviors that are acceptable to the self; that are consistent with one's fundamental personality. *Ego-dystonic* refers to feelings, thoughts, and/or behaviors that are distressing, unacceptable, or inconsistent with one's self-concept.

WARDS TIP

Personality disorder criteria—**CAPRI**

Cognition
Affect
Personal **R**elations
Impulse control

Definition

Personality is one's set of stable, predictable, emotional, and behavioral traits. Personality *disorders* involve enduring patterns of inner experience and behavior that deviate markedly from expectations of an individual's culture. They are pervasive, **maladaptive,** and cause significant impairment in social or occupational functioning. Patients with personality disorders often lack insight about their problems; their symptoms are either **ego-syntonic** or viewed as immutable. In addition, individuals with personality disorders have significant comorbidity with other mental disorders.

DIAGNOSIS AND *DSM-5* CRITERIA

1. Enduring pattern of behavior/inner experience that deviates from the person's culture and is manifested in two or more of the following ways:
   - Cognition
   - Affect
   - Interpersonal functioning
   - Impulse control
2. The pattern:
   - Is **pervasive** and **inflexible** in a broad range of situations.
   - Is **stable** and has an onset no later than adolescence or early adulthood.
   - Leads to significant distress in functioning.
   - Is not accounted for by another mental/medical illness or by use of a substance.

The international prevalence of personality disorders is approximately 7–12%. Personality disorders vary by gender. Many patients with personality disorders will meet the criteria for more than one disorder; they should be classified as having all of the disorders for which they qualify.

Clusters

Personality disorders are divided into the following three clusters:

- **Cluster A**—Schizoid, schizotypal, and paranoid:
  - Patients seem eccentric, peculiar, or withdrawn.
  - Familial association with psychotic disorders.
- **Cluster B—Antisocial, borderline, histrionic, and narcissistic:**
  - Patients seem emotional, dramatic, or inconsistent.
  - Familial association with mood disorders.
- **Cluster C—Avoidant, dependent, and obsessive-compulsive:**
  - Patients seem anxious or fearful.
  - Familial association with anxiety disorders.

Other specified/unspecified personality disorder includes characteristics of a personality disorder that do not meet full criteria for any of the other personality disorders.

ETIOLOGY

■ Biological, genetic, and psychosocial factors during childhood and adolescence contribute to the development of personality disorders.

■ The prevalence of some personality disorders in monozygotic twins is several times higher than in dizygotic twins.

TREATMENT

■ Personality disorders are generally very difficult to treat, especially since few patients are aware that they need help. The disorders tend to be chronic and lifelong.

■ In general, pharmacologic treatment has limited usefulness (see individual exceptions below) except in treating comorbid mental conditions (e.g., major depressive disorder).

■ Psychotherapy is usually the most helpful.

Cluster A

These patients are perceived as eccentric or odd by others and can have psychotic symptoms (see Table 6-1).

PARANOID PERSONALITY DISORDER (PPD)

Patients with PPD have a pervasive distrust and suspiciousness of others and often interpret motives as malevolent. They tend to blame their own problems on others and seem angry and hostile. They are often characterized as being pathologically jealous, which leads them to think that their sexual partners or spouses are cheating on them.

Diagnosis and DSM-5 *Criteria*

■ Diagnosis requires a general distrust of others, beginning by early adulthood and present in a variety of contexts.

TABLE 6-1. Cluster A Personality Disorders and Classic Clinical Examples	
Personality Disorder	Clinical Example
Paranoid personality disorder	A 30-year-old man says his wife has been cheating on him because he does not have a good enough job to provide for her needs. He also claims that on his previous job, his boss laid him off because he did a better job than his boss. He has initiated several lawsuits. He believes the neighbors are critical of him. He refuses couples therapy because he is certain the therapist will side with his wife.
Schizoid personality disorder	A 45-year-old scientist works in the lab most of the day and, according to his coworkers, has no friends. He is at risk of losing this job because of a failure to collaborate with others. He expresses no desire to make friends and is content with his single life. He has no evidence of a thought disorder.
Schizotypal personality disorder	A 35-year-old man dresses in a wizard costume every weekend with friends as part of a live action role-playing community. He spends a great deal of time on his computers set up in his basement for video games and to "detect the presence of extraterrestrial communications in space." He has no auditory or visual hallucinations. He is lonely and sad, feels ostracized by others, and desires an intimate relationship.

- At least four of the following must also be present:
  1. Suspicion (without evidence) that others are exploiting or deceiving them.
  2. Preoccupation with doubts of loyalty or trustworthiness of friends or acquaintances.
  3. Reluctance to confide in others.
  4. Interpretation of benign remarks as threatening or demeaning.
  5. Persistence of grudges.
  6. Perception of attacks on their character that is not apparent to others; quick to counterattack.
  7. Suspicions regarding fidelity of spouse or partner.

Epidemiology

- Prevalence: 1–4%.
- More commonly diagnosed in men than in women.
- Higher incidence in family members of schizophrenics.
- This personality disorder may be misdiagnosed in minority groups, immigrants, and deaf individuals.

Differential Diagnosis

- *Schizophrenia:* Unlike patients with schizophrenia, patients with PPD *do not have any fixed delusions and are not frankly psychotic*, although they may have transient psychosis under stressful situations.
- *Social disenfranchisement and social isolation:* Without a social support system, individuals can react with suspicion to others. The differential in favor of PPD can be assisted by collateral history from others in close contact with the person, who may identify what they consider as excess suspicion.

Course and Prognosis

- The disorder usually has a chronic course, causing lifelong marital and job-related problems.

Treatment

- Psychotherapy is the treatment of choice, although, as stated above, patients rarely initiate treatment.
- Group psychotherapy should be avoided due to mistrust and misinterpretation of others' statements.
- Patients may also benefit from a short course of antipsychotics for transient psychosis.

SCHIZOID PERSONALITY DISORDER

Patients with schizoid personality disorder have a lifelong pattern of social withdrawal. They are often perceived as eccentric and reclusive. They are quiet, unsociable, and have a constricted affect. They have *no desire for close relationships* and prefer to be alone.

Diagnosis and DSM-5 Criteria

- A pattern of voluntary social withdrawal and restricted range of emotional expression, beginning by early adulthood and present in a variety of contexts.
- Four or more of the following must also be present:
  1. Neither enjoying nor desiring close relationships (including family).
  2. Generally choosing solitary activities.
  3. Little (if any) interest in sexual activity with another person.

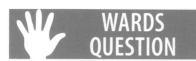

WARDS QUESTION

Q: What is the key difference between schizoid and avoidant personality disorders?
A: Patients with schizoid personality disorder *prefer* to be alone whereas those with avoidant personality disorder prefer to be in a relationship.

4. Taking pleasure in few activities (if any).
5. Few close friends or confidants (if any).
6. Indifference to praise or criticism.
7. Emotional coldness, detachment, or flattened affect.

Epidemiology

- Prevalence: 3–5%.
- Diagnosed more often in men than women.
- May be increased prevalence of schizoid personality disorder in relatives of individuals with schizophrenia.

Differential Diagnosis

- *Schizophrenia:* Unlike patients with schizophrenia, patients with schizoid personality disorder do not have overt psychotic symptoms such as delusions or hallucinations.
- *Schizotypal personality disorder:* Patients with schizoid personality disorder do not have the same eccentric behavior or magical thinking seen in patients with schizotypal personality disorder. Schizotypal patients are more similar to schizophrenic patients in terms of odd perceptions, thought, and behavior.

Course
Usually chronic course.

Treatment

- Lack insight for individual psychotherapy, and may find group therapy threatening; may benefit from day programs or drop-in centers.
- Antidepressants if comorbid major depression is diagnosed.

SCHIZOTYPAL PERSONALITY DISORDER

Patients with schizotypal personality disorder have a pervasive pattern of eccentric behavior and peculiar thought patterns. They are often perceived as strange and odd. The disorder was developed out of the observation that certain family traits predominate in first-degree relatives of those with schizophrenia.

Diagnosis and DSM-5 Criteria

- A pattern of social deficits marked by eccentric behavior, cognitive or perceptual distortions, and discomfort with close relationships, beginning by early adulthood and present in a variety of contexts.
- Five or more of the following must be present:
  1. Ideas of reference (excluding delusions of reference).
  2. Odd beliefs or magical thinking, inconsistent with cultural norms.
  3. Unusual perceptual experiences (such as bodily illusions).
  4. Suspiciousness.
  5. Inappropriate or restricted affect.
  6. Odd or eccentric appearance or behavior.
  7. Few close friends or confidants.
  8. Odd thinking or speech (vague, stereotyped, etc.).
  9. Excessive social anxiety.
- Magical thinking may include:
  - Belief in clairvoyance or telepathy.
  - Bizarre fantasies or preoccupations.
  - Belief in superstitions.
- Odd behaviors may include involvement in cults or strange religious practices.

Epidemiology

Prevalence: 4%.

Differential Diagnosis

- *Schizophrenia:* Unlike patients with schizophrenia, patients with schizotypal personality disorder are not frankly psychotic (though they can become transiently so under stress), nor do they have delusions.
- *Schizoid personality disorder:* Patients with schizoid personality disorder do not have the same eccentric behavior seen in patients with schizotypal personality disorder.

Course

- Course is chronic, with a small minority developing schizophrenia.
- Premorbid personality type for a patient with schizophrenia.

Treatment

- Psychotherapy is the treatment of choice to help develop social skills training.
- A short course of low-dose second-generation antipsychotic may help with the cognitive-perceptual disturbances.

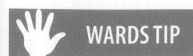

WARDS TIP

Q: What is the premorbid personality seen in schizophrenia?
A: Schizotypal personality disorder.

Cluster B

Includes antisocial, borderline, histrionic, and narcissistic personality disorders. These patients are often emotional, impulsive, and dramatic (Table 6-2).

 Mr. Harris is a 35-year-old man with no prior psychiatric history who was arrested for assaulting his pregnant girlfriend. While in jail, he reports feeling depressed, and you are called in for a psychiatric evaluation. Mr. Harris is cooperative during the evaluation and presents as friendly and likeable. He reports that he is innocent of his charges and expresses feeling sad and tearful since his incarceration 2 days ago. He requests that you transfer him to the mental health unit at the correctional facility. However, you perform a thorough evaluation, and you do not find symptoms suggestive of a mood or psychotic disorder. When asked if he has been incarcerated before, he reports a history of multiple arrests and convictions for robbery and gun possession. He reports that he is unemployed because he has been "in and out of jail" during the past 5 years. He provides rationalizations for his limited involvement in these past crimes and does not appear remorseful.

Mr. Harris reveals a pattern of repeated fights since childhood and says that he quit school while in the ninth grade after being suspended for smoking pot on school grounds. Mr. Harris reports that throughout his childhood he bullied others, and laughs when recounting an episode during which he threw his cat against the wall to see if it would bounce back. He denies any family history of psychiatric illnesses, but reports that his father is currently incarcerated for drug trafficking.

What is his diagnosis?

Mr. Harris's diagnosis is antisocial personality disorder. His history shows a pervasive pattern of disregard for and violation of the rights of others since age 15, and there is evidence of conduct disorder with onset before age 15 years. Remember that, although it is common, not all criminals have antisocial personality disorder.

What are some associated findings?

Antisocial personality disorder is more prevalent in males, is associated with low socioeconomic background, and has a genetic predisposition. It has been found that the children of parents with antisocial personality disorder have an increased risk for this disorder, somatic symptom disorder, and substance use disorders.

TABLE 6-2. Cluster B Personality Disorders and Classic Clinical Examples

Personality Disorder	Clinical Example
Antisocial personality disorder	A 30-year-old unemployed man has been accused of killing three senior citizens after robbing them. He is surprisingly charming in the interview. In his adolescence, he was arrested several times for stealing cars and assaulting other kids.
Borderline personality disorder	A 23-year-old medical student attempted to cut her wrist because things did not work out with a man she had been dating over the past 3 weeks. She states that guys are jerks and "not worth her time." She often feels that she is "alone in this world."
Histrionic personality disorder	A 33-year-old provocatively dressed woman comes to your office complaining that her fever feels like "she is burning in hell." She vividly describes how the fever has affected her work as a teacher but displays superficial expressions of emotion.
Narcissistic personality disorder	A 48-year-old company CEO is rushed to the ED after an automobile accident. He does not let the residents operate on him and requests the Chief of trauma surgery as he is "vital to the company." He makes several business phone calls in the ED to stay on "top of his game."

ANTISOCIAL PERSONALITY DISORDER

Patients diagnosed with antisocial personality disorder often exploit and violate the rights of others, and break rules to meet their own needs. They lack empathy, compassion, and remorse for their actions. They are impulsive, deceitful, and often violate the law. They are frequently skilled at reading social cues and can appear charming and normal to others who meet them for the first time and do not know their history.

Diagnosis and DSM-5 Criteria

- Pattern of disregard for and violation of the rights of others since age 15.
- Patients must be **at least 18 years old** for this diagnosis; history of behavior as a child/adolescent must be consistent with **conduct disorder** (see Chapter 10, "Psychiatric Disorders in Children").
- Three or more of the following should be present:
  1. Failure to conform to social norms by committing unlawful acts.
  2. Deceitfulness/repeated lying/manipulating others for personal gain.
  3. Impulsivity/failure to plan ahead.
  4. Irritability and aggressiveness/repeated fights or assaults.
  5. Recklessness and disregard for safety of self or others.
  6. Irresponsibility/failure to sustain work or honor financial obligations.
  7. Lack of remorse for actions.

Epidemiology

- Prevalence: 1–4% of the general population.
- Males are three to five times as likely to be diagnosed as women.
- Males with alcoholic parents are at increased risk.
- There is a higher incidence in poor urban areas and in prisoners but no racial difference.
- Genetic component: Increased risk among first-degree relatives.

Differential Diagnosis

Substance use disorder: It is necessary to ascertain which came first. Patients who began abusing drugs before their antisocial behavior started may have behavior attributable to the effects of their addiction.

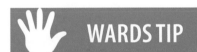

WARDS TIP

Symptoms of antisocial personality disorder—**CORRUPT**
Cannot follow law
Obligations ignored
Remorselessness
Reckless disregard for safety
Underhanded (deceitful)
Planning deficit (impulsive)
Temper (irritable, aggressive)

KEY FACT

Antisocial personality disorder begins in childhood as conduct disorder. Patient may have a history of being abused (physically or sexually) as a child or a history of hurting animals or starting fires. It is often associated with violations of the law.

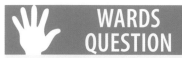

WARDS QUESTION

Q: What is the most commonly diagnosed personality disorder in psychiatric inpatients?
A: Borderline personality disorder.

WARDS TIP

Symptoms of BPD—**IMPULSIVE**
Impulsive
Moody
Paranoid under stress
Unstable self-image
Labile, intense relationships
Suicidal
Inappropriate anger
Vulnerable to abandonment
Emptiness

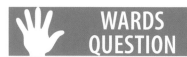

WARDS QUESTION

Q: What is a common defense mechanism used by patients with BPD?
A: *Splitting*—They view others and themselves as all good or all bad.

Course

- Usually has a chronic course, but some improvement of symptoms may occur as the patient ages.
- Many patients have multiple somatic complaints, and coexistence of substance use disorders and/or major depression is common.
- There is increased morbidity from substance use, trauma, suicide, or homicide.

Treatment

- Psychotherapy is generally ineffective.
- Pharmacotherapy may be used to treat symptoms of anxiety, depression, or aggression, but use caution given the high comorbidity with substance use disorders in these patients.

BORDERLINE PERSONALITY DISORDER (BPD)

Patients with BPD have unstable moods, behaviors, and interpersonal relationships. They fear abandonment and have poorly formed identity. Relationships begin with intense attachments and end with the slightest conflict. Aggression is common. They are impulsive and may have a history of repeated suicide attempts/gestures or episodes of self-mutilation. They have higher rates of childhood physical, emotional, and sexual abuse than the general population.

Diagnosis and DSM-5 Criteria

- Pervasive pattern of impulsivity and unstable relationships, affects, self-image, and behaviors, present by early adulthood and in a variety of contexts.
- At least five of the following must be present:
  1. Frantic efforts to avoid real or imagined abandonment.
  2. Unstable, intense interpersonal relationships (e.g., extreme love–hate relationships).
  3. Unstable self-image.
  4. Impulsivity in at least two potentially harmful ways (spending, sexual activity, substance use, binge eating, etc.).
  5. Recurrent suicidal threats or attempts or self-mutilation.
  6. Unstable mood/affect.
  7. Chronic feelings of emptiness.
  8. Difficulty controlling anger.
  9. Transient, stress-related paranoid ideation or dissociative symptoms.

Epidemiology

- Lifetime prevalence: 6%.
- Diagnosed three times more often in women than men in clinical settings.
- Suicide rate: 10%.

Differential Diagnosis

- *Schizophrenia:* Unlike patients with schizophrenia, patients with BPD do not have frank psychosis (may have transient psychosis, however, if they decompensate under stress or substances of abuse).
- *Bipolar I/II:* Mood swings experienced in BPD are rapid, brief, moment-to-moment reactions to perceived environmental or psychological triggers.

Course

- Variable, but many develop stability in middle age.
- High incidence of coexisting major depression and/or substance use disorders.
- Increased risk of suicide.

Treatment

- Dialectical behavior therapy (DBT) is the treatment of choice—includes cognitive-behavioral therapy, mindfulness skills, and group therapy.
- Other psychotherapies found to be beneficial include mentalization-based therapy, transference-focused therapy, and schema-focused therapy.
- Pharmacotherapy should be considered an adjunct to psychotherapy. Mood stabilizers and low-dose antipsychotic medications have been found to be more effective than antidepressants in the treatment of mood swings/lability.

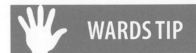

WARDS TIP

Pharmacotherapy has been shown to be more useful in BPD than in any other personality disorder.

HISTRIONIC PERSONALITY DISORDER (HPD)

Patients with HPD exhibit attention-seeking behavior and excessive emotionality. They are dramatic, flamboyant, and extroverted, but are unable to form long-lasting, meaningful relationships. They are often sexually inappropriate and provocative.

Diagnosis and DSM-5 Criteria

- Pattern of excessive emotionality and attention seeking, present by early adulthood and in a variety of contexts.
- At least five of the following must be present:
  1. Uncomfortable when not the center of attention.
  2. Inappropriately seductive or provocative behavior.
  3. Rapidly shifting but shallow expression of emotion.
  4. Uses physical appearance to draw attention to self.
  5. Speech that is impressionistic and lacking in detail.
  6. Theatrical and exaggerated expression of emotion.
  7. Easily influenced by others or situation.
  8. Perceives relationships as more intimate than they actually are.

Epidemiology

- Prevalence in the general population: <2%.
- Women are more likely to have HPD than men.

Differential Diagnosis

BPD: Patients with BPD are more likely to suffer from depression, brief psychotic episodes, and to attempt suicide. HPD patients are generally more functional.

Course

Usually chronic, with some improvement of symptoms with age.

Treatment

- Psychotherapy (e.g., supportive, problem-solving, interpersonal, group) is the treatment of choice.
- Pharmacotherapy to treat associated depressive or anxious symptoms as necessary.

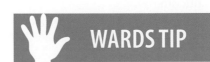

WARDS TIP

Histrionic patients often use the defense mechanism of *regression*—they revert to childlike behaviors.

NARCISSISTIC PERSONALITY DISORDER (NPD)

Patients with NPD have a sense of superiority, a need for admiration, and a lack of empathy. They consider themselves "special" and will exploit others for their own gain. Despite their grandiosity, however, these patients often have fragile self-esteem.

Diagnosis and DSM-5 Criteria

- Pattern of grandiosity, need for admiration, and lack of empathy beginning by early adulthood and present in a variety of contexts.
- Five or more of the following must be present:
  1. Exaggerated sense of self-importance.
  2. Preoccupation with fantasies of unlimited money, success, brilliance, etc.
  3. Believe that they are "special" or unique and can associate only with other high-status individuals.
  4. Requires excessive admiration.
  5. Has sense of entitlement.
  6. Takes advantage of others for self-gain.
  7. Lacks empathy.
  8. Envious of others or believes others are envious of them.
  9. Arrogant or haughty.

Epidemiology
Prevalence: Approximately 6%.

Differential Diagnosis
Antisocial personality disorder: Both types of patients exploit others, but NPD patients want status and recognition, while antisocial patients want material gain or simply the subjugation of others. Narcissistic patients become depressed when they don't get the recognition they think they deserve.

Course
Usually has a chronic course; higher incidence of depression and midlife crises since these patients put such a high value on youth and power.

Treatment
- Psychotherapy is the treatment of choice.
- Psychotropics may be used if a comorbid psychiatric disorder is also diagnosed.

Cluster C

Includes avoidant, dependent, and obsessive-compulsive personality disorders. These patients appear anxious and fearful (see Table 6-3).

AVOIDANT PERSONALITY DISORDER

Patients with avoidant personality disorder have a pervasive pattern of social inhibition and an intense fear of rejection. They will avoid situations in which they may be rejected. Their fear of rejection is so overwhelming that it affects all aspects of their lives. They avoid social interactions and may seek jobs in which there is little interpersonal contact. These patients *desire* companionship but are extremely shy and easily injured.

WARDS TIP

Narcissism is characterized by an inflated sense of entitlement. People with narcissistic personality are often "fishing for compliments" and become irritated and anxious when they are not treated as important.

WARDS QUESTION

Q: Which personality disorder has an overlap with social anxiety disorder (social phobia)?
A: Avoidant personality disorder (may be same syndrome/spectrum).

WARDS TIP

Symptoms of avoidant personality disorder—**AFRAID**

Avoids occupation with others
Fear of embarrassment and criticism
Reserved unless they are certain that they are liked
Always thinking rejection
Isolates from relationships
Distances self unless certain that they are liked

TABLE 6-3. Cluster C Personality Disorders and Classic Clinical Examples	
Personality Disorder	**Clinical Example**
Avoidant personality disorder	A 30-year-old postal worker rarely goes out with her coworkers and often makes excuses when they ask her to join them because she is afraid they will not like her. She wishes to go out and meet new people but, according to her, she is too "shy."
Dependent personality disorder	A 40-year-old man who lives with his parents has trouble deciding how to get his car fixed. He calls his father at work several times to ask very trivial things. He has been unemployed over the past 3 years. He has been in several long-term but abusive relationships.
Obsessive-compulsive personality disorder	A 40-year-old secretary has been recently fired because of her inability to prepare some work projects in time. According to her, they were not in the right format and she had to revise them six times, which led to the delay. This has happened before but she feels that she is not given enough time to "get it perfect."

Diagnosis and DSM-5 Criteria

- A pattern of social inhibition, hypersensitivity, and feelings of inadequacy since early adulthood.
- At least four of the following must be present:
  1. Avoids occupation that involves interpersonal contact due to a fear of criticism and rejection.
  2. Unwilling to interact unless certain of being liked.
  3. Cautious of interpersonal relationships.
  4. Preoccupied with being criticized or rejected in social situations.
  5. Inhibited in new social situations because he or she feels inadequate.
  6. Believes they are socially inept and inferior.
  7. Reluctant to engage in new activities for fear of embarrassment.

Epidemiology

- Prevalence: Approximately 2%.

Differential Diagnosis

- *Schizoid personality disorder:* Patients with avoidant personality disorder desire companionship but are extremely shy, whereas patients with schizoid personality disorder have little or no desire for companionship.
- *Social anxiety disorder (social phobia):* See Chapter 5, "Anxiety Obsessive-Compulsive, Trauma, and Stressor-Related Disorders." Both involve fear and avoidance of social situations. If the symptoms are an integral part of the patient's personality and have been evident since adolescence, personality disorder is the more likely diagnosis. Social anxiety disorder involves a fear of *embarrassment* in a particular setting (speaking in public, urinating in public, etc.), whereas avoidant personality disorder is an overall fear of *rejection* and a sense of inadequacy. However, a patient can have both disorders concurrently and should carry both diagnoses if criteria for each are met.
- *Dependent personality disorder:* Avoidant personality disorder patients cling to relationships, similar to dependent personality disorder patients; however, avoidant patients are slow to get involved, whereas dependent patients actively and aggressively seek relationships.

 KEY FACT

Schizoid patients *prefer* to be alone. Avoidant patients want to be with others but are too scared of rejection.

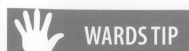

WARDS TIP

Symptoms of dependent personality disorder—**OBEDIENT**

Obsessive about approval
Bound by other's decisions
Enterprises are rarely initiated due to their lack of self-confidence
Difficult to make own decisions
Invalid feelings while alone
Engrossed with fears of self-reliance
Needs to be in a relationship
Tentative about decisions

KEY FACT

Regression is often seen in people with DPD. This is defined as going back to a younger age of maturity.

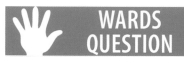

WARDS QUESTION

Q: What childhood conditions predispose to later development of DPD?
A: Medical illness and separation anxiety disorders.

Course

- Course is usually chronic, although may remit with age.
- Particularly difficult during adolescence, when attractiveness and socialization are important.
- Increased incidence of associated anxiety and depressive disorders.
- If support system fails, patient is left very susceptible to depression, anxiety, and anger.

Treatment

- Psychotherapy, including assertiveness and social skills training, is most effective.
- Group therapy may also be beneficial.
- Selective serotonin reuptake inhibitors (SSRIs) may be prescribed for comorbid social anxiety disorder or major depression.

DEPENDENT PERSONALITY DISORDER (DPD)

Patients with DPD have poor self-confidence and fear of separation. They have an excessive need to be taken care of and allow others to make decisions for them. They feel helpless when left alone.

Diagnosis and DSM-5 Criteria

- A pattern of excessive need to be taken care of that leads to submissive and clinging behavior.
- At least five of the following must be present:
  1. Difficulty making everyday decisions without reassurance from others.
  2. Need others to assume responsibilities for most areas of their life.
  3. Difficulty expressing disagreement because of fear of loss of approval.
  4. Difficulty initiating projects because of lack of self-confidence.
  5. Goes to excessive lengths to obtain support from others.
  6. Feels helpless when alone.
  7. Urgently seeks another relationship when one ends.
  8. Preoccupied with fears of being left to take care of self.

Epidemiology

- Prevalence: Approximately 2%.
- Women are more likely to be diagnosed with DPD than men.
- Childhood medical illness or separation anxiety disorder may increase the likelihood of developing DPD.

Differential Diagnosis

- *Avoidant personality disorder:* See discussion above.
- *BPD and HPD:* Patients with DPD usually have a long-lasting relationship with one person on whom they are dependent. While patients with borderline and histrionic personality disorders are often dependent on other people, they are unable to maintain long-lasting relationships.

Course

- Usually has a chronic course.
- Patients are prone to depression, particularly after loss of person on whom they are dependent.
- Difficulties with employment since they cannot act independently or without close supervision.

Treatment

- Psychotherapy, particularly cognitive-behavioral, assertiveness, and social skills training, is the treatment of choice.
- Pharmacotherapy may be used to treat associated symptoms of anxiety or depression.

OBSESSIVE-COMPULSIVE PERSONALITY DISORDER (OCPD)

Patients with OCPD have a pervasive pattern of perfectionism, inflexibility, and orderliness. They become so preoccupied with unimportant details that they are often unable to complete simple tasks in a timely fashion. They appear stiff, serious, and formal, with constricted affect. They are often successful professionally but have poor interpersonal skills.

Diagnosis and DSM-5 Criteria

- Pattern of preoccupation with orderliness, control, and perfectionism at the expense of efficiency and flexibility, present by early adulthood and in a variety of contexts.
- At least four of the following must be present:
  1. Preoccupation with details, rules, lists, and organization such that the major point of the activity is lost.
  2. Perfectionism that is detrimental to completion of task.
  3. Excessive devotion to work.
  4. Excessive conscientiousness and scrupulousness about morals and ethics.
  5. Will not delegate tasks.
  6. Unable to discard worthless objects.
  7. Miserly spending style.
  8. Rigid and stubborn.

Epidemiology

- Prevalence: 2–7%.
- Men are two times more likely to be diagnosed with OCPD than women.

Differential Diagnosis

- *Obsessive-compulsive disorder (OCD):* Patients with OCPD do not have the recurrent obsessions or compulsions that are present in OCD. In addition, the symptoms of OCPD are **ego-syntonic** rather than ego-dystonic (as in OCD); OCD patients are aware that they have a problem and wish that their thoughts and behaviors would go away.
- *NPD:* Both disorders entail assertiveness and achievement, but NPD patients are motivated by status, whereas OCPD patients are motivated by perfectionism and the work itself.

Course

- Unpredictable course.
- A significant number have comorbid OCD (most do not, however).

Treatment

- Psychotherapy is the treatment of choice. Cognitive-behavior therapy may be particularly useful.
- Pharmacotherapy may be used to treat associated symptoms as necessary.

PERSONALITY CHANGE DUE TO ANOTHER MEDICAL CONDITION

This refers to a persistent personality change from a previous pattern due to the direct pathophysiological result of a medical condition (e.g., head trauma, stroke, epilepsy, central nervous system infection, or neoplasm). Subtypes include labile, disinhibited, aggressive, apathetic, or paranoid.

OTHER SPECIFIED PERSONALITY DISORDER

This diagnosis is reserved for a personality disorder that does not meet the full criteria for any of the disorders, but where the clinician *chooses* to communicate the specific reason that the presentation does not meet the criteria for any specific personality disorder (e.g., "mixed personality disorder").

UNSPECIFIED PERSONALITY DISORDER

This diagnosis is used for a personality disorder that does not meet the full criteria for any of the disorders, but where the clinician chooses *not* to specify the reason that the criteria are not met for any specific personality disorder (e.g., not enough information to make a more specific diagnosis).

Substance Use Disorders

Substance use disorders are characterized by a problematic pattern of substance use that leads to some form of functional impairment or distress. Keep in mind that frequent use of a substance does not necessarily indicate a *substance use disorder* unless it is causing problems for the patient.

DIAGNOSIS AND *DSM-5* CRITERIA

Substance use disorders are characterized by a problematic pattern of substance use causing impairment or distress, as manifested by at least two of the following within a 12-month period:

- Using substance more than originally intended.
- Persistent desire or unsuccessful efforts to cut down on use.
- Significant time spent in obtaining, using, or recovering from substance.
- Craving to use substance.
- Failure to fulfill obligations at work, school, or home.
- Continued use despite social or interpersonal problems due to the substance use.
- Limiting social, occupational, or recreational activities because of substance use.
- Use in dangerous situations (e.g., driving a car).
- Continued use despite subsequent physical or psychological problem (e.g., drinking alcohol despite worsening liver problems).
- Tolerance (needing higher amounts of the substance to achieve the desired effect *or* experiencing diminished effects when repeating the same dose).
- Withdrawal (a substance-specific syndrome occurring when a patient stops or reduces heavy/prolonged substance use).

Note that these criteria remain the same regardless of what substance(s) the patient is using. The disorder may be classified as mild, moderate, or severe depending on the number of criteria met.

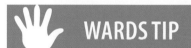

WARDS TIP

It is possible to have a substance use disorder without having physiological dependence (i.e., without having withdrawal or tolerance).

EPIDEMIOLOGY

- One-year prevalence of any substance use disorder in the United States is approximately 8%.
- More common in men than women.
- Alcohol and nicotine are the most commonly used substances.

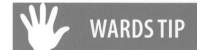

WARDS TIP

Substance-induced mood symptoms improve during prolonged abstinence, whereas *primary* mood symptoms persist.

PSYCHIATRIC SYMPTOMS

- Mood symptoms are common among persons with substance use disorders.
- Psychotic symptoms may occur with some substances.
- Personality disorders and psychiatric comorbidities (e.g., major depression, anxiety disorders) are common among persons with substance use disorders.
- It is often challenging to decide whether psychiatric symptoms are primary or substance-induced. Many patients may use substances to self-medicate for undertreated psychiatric symptoms.

KEY FACT

Withdrawal symptoms of a drug are usually the opposite of its intoxication effects. For example, alcohol is sedating, but alcohol *withdrawal* can cause brain excitation and seizures.

ACUTE INTOXICATION AND WITHDRAWAL

Both the intoxicated and withdrawing patient can present difficulties in diagnosis and treatment. Since it is common for persons to abuse several substances at once, the clinical presentation is often confusing, and signs/symptoms may be atypical. Always be on the lookout for use of multiple substances.

DETECTION OF SUBSTANCE USE

See Table 7-1.

TREATMENT OF SUBSTANCE USE DISORDERS

- Behavioral counseling should be part of every substance use disorder treatment.
See Table 7-2.

- Psychosocial treatments are effective and include motivational intervention (MI), cognitive-behavioral therapy (CBT), contingency management, and individual and group therapy.

- For severe substance use disorders, residential (usually 28-day) "rehab" programs are common; some patients may choose to do partial hospitalization or intensive outpatient programming.

TABLE 7-1. Direct Testing for Substance Use	
Alcohol	■ Stays in system for only a few hours. ■ Breathalyzer test, commonly used by law enforcement. ■ Blood/urine testing more accurate. ■ Urine screening for metabolite (ethyl glucuronide) — not useful for assessing acute intoxication, but can indicate alcohol use over the preceding 2–5 days.
Cocaine	■ Urine drug screen positive for 2–4 days (up to 8 days for heavy users).
Amphetamines	■ Urine drug screen positive for 1–3 days. ■ Most assays have poor sensitivity and/or specificity.
Phencyclidine (PCP)	■ Urine drug screen positive for 4–7 days. ■ OTC cold medications may yield false positive. ■ Creatine kinase (CK) and aspartate aminotransferase (AST) are often elevated.
Sedative-hypnotics	In urine and blood for variable amounts of time. *Barbiturates:* ■ Short-acting (pentobarbital): 24 hours ■ Long-acting (phenobarbital): 3 weeks *Benzodiazepines:* ■ Short-acting (e.g., lorazepam): up to 5 days ■ Long-acting (diazepam): up to 30 days
Opioids	■ Urine drug test remains positive for 1–3 days, depending on opioid used. ■ Routine screening tests detect morphine, which is the eventual metabolite of all natural opioids. ■ Buprenorphine, synthetic opioids (methadone, fentanyl, tramadol) and semi-synthetic opioids (oxycodone, hydrocodone) will not be detected on routine screening (order separate assay).
Marijuana	Urine detection: ■ After a single use, about 3 days. In heavy users, up to 4 weeks (THC is released from adipose stores).

TABLE 7-2. Stages of Change		
Stage	Definition	Example
Precontemplation	Patients do not view their addiction as a problem. They may see substance use as helpful and/or enjoyable.	A college student who drinks heavily feels that they need alcohol to overcome social anxiety and enjoy parties. They do not identify any negative consequences from their use.
Contemplation	The patient begins to think about cutting down or stopping altogether. They recognize potential benefits of making a change, but may be ambivalent or feel unable to do so.	The student misses several deadlines due to hangovers from drinking the night before. They think cutting down on alcohol might improve their grades, but aren't sure they want to stop.
Preparation	The patient plans for the process of change. They collect information, and may experiment with very small changes.	The student begins researching self-help strategies for reducing alcohol intake. They look up campus resources for individual and group therapy.
Action	The patient takes direct steps toward reducing or stopping substance use.	The student begins attending substance-use-focused groups on campus, and talks with their primary care doctor about starting naltrexone.
Maintenance	The patient has successfully made significant behavior change, and works to avoid relapse.	The student continues to drink, but limits themself to 1–2 drinks per day, and only consumes alcohol on weekends.
Relapse	After a successful period of remission, patients resume substance use (or fall back into unhealthy patterns of use).	After graduating, the student is unemployed. They begin drinking again to cope with stress and unstructured time, and quickly escalates to near daily use.

- Community-based groups such as SMART Recovery, Alcoholics Anonymous (AA), and Narcotics Anonymous (NA) should also be encouraged as part of the treatment.
- Pharmacotherapy is available for some drugs of abuse, and will be discussed later in this chapter as relevant to a particular substance.

Alcohol (EtOH)

- Alcohol activates gamma-aminobutyric acid (GABA), dopamine, and serotonin receptors in the central nervous system (CNS). It inhibits glutamate receptor activity and voltage-gated calcium channels. GABA receptors are inhibitory, and glutamate receptors are excitatory; thus, alcohol is a potent CNS depressant.
- Lifetime prevalence of alcohol use disorder in the United States is 5% of women and 12% of men.
- Alcohol is metabolized in the following manner:
  1. Alcohol → acetaldehyde (enzyme: *alcohol dehydrogenase*).
  2. Acetaldehyde → acetic acid (enzyme: *aldehyde dehydrogenase*).

These enzymes are upregulated in heavy drinkers. Some populations produce less aldehyde dehydrogenase due to genetic variation, resulting in flushing and nausea with alcohol use.

INTOXICATION

Clinical Presentation

- The absorption and elimination rates of alcohol are variable and depend on many factors, including age, sex, body weight, chronic nature of use,

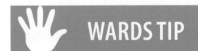 **WARDS TIP**

Alcohol is the most common co-ingestant in drug overdoses.

 KEY FACT

Most adults will show some signs of intoxication with BAL >100 and obvious signs with BAL >150 mg/dL.

WARDS QUESTION

Q: What is the average rate of alcohol metabolism?
A: Between 15 and 35 mg/dL per hour.

KEY FACT

Ethanol, along with methanol and ethylene glycol, can be a cause of anion gap metabolic acidosis.

KEY FACT

Males with substance use disorders, especially alcohol, have higher rates of perpetrating domestic violence.

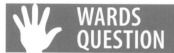

WARDS QUESTION

Q: What are the typical features of Wernicke's encephalopathy?
A: The classic triad is confusion (altered mental status), ataxic gait, and oculomotor findings (typically nystagmus or gaze palsies).

TABLE 7-3. Clinical Presentation of Alcohol Intoxication	
Effects	**BAL**
Impaired fine motor control	20–50 mg/dL
Impaired judgment and coordination	50–100 mg/dL
Ataxic gait and poor balance	100–150 mg/dL
Lethargy, difficulty sitting upright, difficulty with memory, nausea/vomiting	150–250 mg/dL
Coma (in the novice drinker)	300 mg/dL
Respiratory depression, death possible	400 mg/dL

duration of consumption, food in the stomach, and the state of nutrition and liver health.

- In addition to the above factors, the effects of EtOH also depend on the blood alcohol level (BAL). Serum EtOH level or an expired air breathalyzer can determine the extent of intoxication. As shown in Table 7-3, patients with high tolerance may show diminished effects at a given BAL.

Treatment

- **Monitor:** Airway, breathing, circulation, glucose, electrolytes, acid–base status.
- Give parenteral **thiamine** (to prevent or treat Wernicke's encephalopathy) and folate. Remember thiamine must be given before glucose, as it's a necessary cofactor for glucose metabolism.
- **Naloxone** may be necessary to reverse effects of co-ingested opioids.
- A computed tomography (CT) scan of the head may be necessary to rule out subdural hematoma or other brain injury.
- The liver will eventually metabolize alcohol without any other interventions.
- Severely intoxicated patients may require mechanical ventilation with attention to acid–base balance, temperature, and electrolytes while they are recovering.
- Gastrointestinal evacuation (e.g., gastric lavage, induction of emesis, and charcoal) is not indicated in the treatment of EtOH overdose unless a significant amount of EtOH was ingested within the preceding 30–60 minutes.

WITHDRAWAL

A 42-year-old man has routine surgery for a knee injury. After 72 hours in the hospital he becomes anxious, flushed, diaphoretic, hypertensive, and tachycardic. *What most likely accounts for this patient's symptoms?* Alcohol withdrawal. *Treatment?* Benzodiazepines (chlordiazepoxide [Librium] or lorazepam [Ativan] are considered the drugs of choice). *What are you most concerned about?* Seizures, delirium tremens, autonomic instability, and cardiac arrhythmias. Remember that alcohol withdrawal can be fatal.

Chronic alcohol use has a depressant effect on the CNS, and cessation of use causes a compensatory hyperactivity with glutamate excitotoxicity. Alcohol withdrawal is ***potentially lethal!***

Clinical Presentation

- Signs and symptoms of **alcohol withdrawal syndrome** include insomnia, anxiety, hand tremor, irritability, anorexia, nausea, vomiting, autonomic hyperactivity (diaphoresis, tachycardia, hypertension), psychomotor agitation, fever, seizures, hallucinations, and delirium tremens (see Table 7-4).
- The earliest symptoms of EtOH withdrawal begin between 6 and 24 hours after the patient's last drink and depend on the duration and quantity of EtOH consumption, liver size, and body mass.
- Generalized tonic-clonic seizures usually occur between 12 and 48 hours after cessation of drinking, with a peak around 12–24 hours.
- About a third of persons with seizures develop delirium tremens (DTs).
- Hypomagnesemia may predispose to seizures; thus, it should be corrected promptly.
- Seizures are treated with benzodiazepines. Long-term treatment with anticonvulsants is not recommended for alcohol withdrawal seizures.

Delirium Tremens

- The most serious form of EtOH withdrawal.
- Usually begins 48–96 hours after the last drink but may occur later.
- While only 5% of patients who experience EtOH withdrawal develop DTs, there is a roughly 5% mortality rate (up to 35% if left untreated).
- Physical illness predisposes to the condition.
- Age >30 and prior DTs increase the risk.
- In addition to delirium, symptoms of DTs may include hallucinations (most commonly visual), agitation, gross tremor, autonomic instability, and fluctuating levels of psychomotor activity.
- It is a medical emergency and should be treated with adequate doses of benzodiazepines.

Treatment

- Benzodiazepines (lorazepam, diazepam, or chlordiazepoxide) should be given in sufficient doses to keep the patient calm and lightly sedated, then tapered down slowly. Carbamazepine or valproic acid can be used in mild withdrawal.

KEY FACT

Risk of suicide attempts is higher among those with psychiatric disorders and concurrent substance use (especially alcohol).

KEY FACT

Delirium tremens is a dangerous form of alcohol withdrawal involving mental status and neurological changes. Symptoms include disorientation, agitation, visual and tactile hallucinations, and autonomic instability (increase in respiratory rate, heart rate, and blood pressure). It carries a 5% mortality rate but occurs in only 5% of patients that experience EtOH withdrawal. Patients often require ICU level of care; treatment includes supportive care and benzodiazepines.

TABLE 7-4. Timing of Alcohol Withdrawal Symptoms		
Syndrome	**Clinical Findings**	**Onset After Last Drink**
Minor withdrawal	Tremulousness, mild anxiety, headache, diaphoresis, palpitations, anorexia, gastrointestinal upset; normal mental status	6 to 36 hours
Seizures	Single or brief flurry of generalized tonic-clonic seizures, short postictal period, status epilepticus rare	6 to 48 hours
Alcoholic hallucinosis	Visual, auditory, and/or tactile hallucinations with intact orientation and normal vital signs	12 to 48 hours
Delirium tremens	Delirium, agitation, tachycardia, hypertension, fever, diaphoresis	48 to 96 hours

Source: Used, with permission, from Hoffman RS, Weinhouse GL. Management of moderate and severe alcohol withdrawal syndromes. https://www.uptodate.com/contents/management-of-moderate-and-severe-alcohol-withdrawal-syndromes. © 2021 UpToDate, Inc. and/or its affiliates. All Rights Reserved.

- Parenteral thiamine, folic acid, and a multivitamin to treat nutritional deficiencies ("banana bag").
- Electrolyte and fluid abnormalities must be corrected.
- Monitor withdrawal signs and symptoms with the Clinical Institute Withdrawal Assessment (CIWA) scale.
- Providers must pay careful attention to the level of consciousness, and consider the possibility of traumatic injuries.
- Check for signs of hepatic failure (e.g., ascites, jaundice, caput medusae, coagulopathy).

Alcoholic Ketoacidosis

- Frequently seen in the setting of alcohol cessation after an alcohol binge secondary to protracted vomiting and lack of oral intake.
- Hallmark is ketosis without hyperglycemia and a negative alcohol level.
- Laboratory studies reveal a high anion gap metabolic acidosis, ketonemia, and low levels of potassium, magnesium, and phosphorus.
- Treatment consists of hydration with D5NS, and replacing electrolytes.

KEY FACT

Confabulation—inventing stories of events that never occurred—is often associated with Korsakoff's "psychosis," or alcohol-induced neurocognitive disorder. Patients are unaware that they are "making things up."

Mr. Smith is a 42-year-old divorced man who arrives to the ED requesting treatment for alcohol detoxification. He began drinking at the age of 17. Although he initially drank only on the weekends, his alcohol use gradually progressed to drinking half a pint of whiskey daily by the age of 35. At that time, he arrived to his workplace intoxicated on several occasions and was referred to a 45-day inpatient alcohol addiction program. After completing the program, he was able to maintain sobriety for 7 years. However, 2 years ago he got divorced, was laid off from work, and ultimately relapsed into alcohol use.

Mr. Smith is currently living with his older sister and states that his drinking is "out of control." He had a DUI recently and has a court date in 2 weeks. He has tried to quit alcohol on his own on several occasions. However, when he stops drinking he feels "shaky, sweaty, anxious, and irritable" and thus resumes his alcohol intake. He also reports a history of a seizure 10 years ago, after he abruptly discontinued his alcohol use for a few days.

Mr. Smith's last drink was about 8 hours prior to his arrival at the ED. During the last month he has been feeling sad, with low energy, difficulty falling and staying asleep, low appetite, and difficulty concentrating. He denies suicidal ideation but has significant guilt over not being able to stop drinking. He denies a history of depression or anxiety, and has not received any other psychiatric treatment in the past.

Upon presentation to ER the patient's blood alcohol level was 110, he did not have symptoms of intoxication, and his urine drug screen was negative. Vital signs were significant for blood pressure of 150/90 and pulse of 110 bpm. Complete blood count and electrolytes were within normal limits.

What is Mr. Smith's most likely diagnosis?

The patient has a diagnosis of alcohol use disorder, with current signs of withdrawal. It is clear that he has exhibited symptoms of tolerance and withdrawal, has been using more alcohol than intended, and has made unsuccessful efforts to cut down. He also describes symptoms suggestive of a depressive disorder. The fact that his depressive symptoms began while abusing alcohol warrants a diagnosis of alcohol-induced depressive disorder. However, major depressive disorder should be ruled out once he remits his alcohol use. If his depressive symptoms are indeed substance-induced, they will improve and resolve with continuing sobriety.

> **What would be the next step in management?**
> Given the Mr. Smith's heavy chronic alcohol use and history of complicated withdrawal (i.e., seizure), he should be admitted to an inpatient unit for close monitoring. Outpatient detoxification is not appropriate in this case. He will likely require a standing and PRN benzodiazepine (the particular benzodiazepine sometimes varies depending on hospital's protocol), as well as close monitoring for signs of withdrawal.

ALCOHOL USE DISORDER

- The **AUDIT-C** (Table 7-5) is used to screen for alcohol use disorder.
- Biochemical markers are useful in detecting recent prolonged drinking; ongoing monitoring of biomarkers can also help detect a relapse. Most commonly used biomarkers are BAL, liver function tests ([LFTs]—aspartate aminotransferase [AST], alanine aminotransferase [ALT]), gamma-glutamyl transpeptidase (GGT), and mean corpuscular volume (MCV). Urine screening for ethyl glucuronide can indicate alcohol use in the 2–5 days prior to testing.

Medications for Alcohol Use Disorder
See Table 7-6.

Long-Term Complications of Alcohol Intake

- **Wernicke's encephalopathy:**
  - Caused by thiamine (vitamin B1) deficiency resulting from poor nutrition.

WARDS TIP

At-risk or heavy drinking for men is more than 4 drinks per day or more than 14 drinks per week. For women, it is more than 3 drinks per day or more than 7 drinks per week.

KEY FACT

AST:ALT ratio ≥2:1 and elevated GGT suggest excessive long-term alcohol use; they take a few weeks to return to normal during abstinence.

TABLE 7-5. AUDIT-C	
Question #1: How often did you have a drink containing alcohol in the past year?	
■ Never	(0 points)
■ Monthly or less	(1 point)
■ Two to four times a month	(2 points)
■ Two to three times per week	(3 points)
■ Four or more times a week	(4 points)
Question #2: How many drinks did you have on a typical day when you were drinking in the past year?	
■ 1 or 2	(0 points)
■ 3 or 4	(1 point)
■ 5 or 6	(2 points)
■ 7 to 9	(3 points)
■ 10 or more	(4 points)
Question #3: How often did you have six or more drinks on one occasion in the past year?	
■ Never	(0 points)
■ Less than monthly	(1 point)
■ Monthly	(2 points)
■ Weekly	(3 points)
■ Daily or almost daily	(4 points)

The AUDIT-C is scored on a scale of 0–12 (scores of 0 reflect no alcohol use). In men, a score of 4 or more is considered positive; in women, a score of 3 or more is considered positive.

TABLE 7-6. Pharmacological Treatment of Alcohol Use Disorder

Medication	Mechanism	Pros	Cons
Naltrexone	Opioid receptor antagonist; reduces cravings and the "high" associated with alcohol intoxication.	First-line treatment. Available as an oral tablet (can be taken daily, or as-needed on drinking days), or monthly injection. Can allow some patients to engage in moderate alcohol use without escalating to binge drinking.	Will precipitate withdrawal in patients with physical opioid dependence. Can interfere with anesthesia (e.g., for acute injury or planned surgeries). Risk of LFT elevation.
Acamprosate	Likely modulates glutamate transmission.	First-line treatment. Can be used for patients with liver disease. Typically used for relapse prevention in patients who have already stopped drinking.	Contraindicated in severe renal disease.
Disulfiram	Blocks aldehyde dehydrogenase, causing buildup of acetaldehyde and aversive symptoms (flushing, headache, nausea/vomiting, palpitations, shortness of breath).	Second-line. Can be effective for highly motivated patients.	Medication adherence can be an issue. Contraindicated in severe cardiac disease, pregnancy, psychosis. Must monitor LFTs.
Topiramate	Anticonvulsant; potentiates GABA and inhibits glutamate receptors.	Second-line treatment. Reduces cravings for alcohol, and decreases alcohol use.	Common adverse effects: impaired cognition ("DOPE-a-max"), nausea / weight loss, metabolic acidosis.

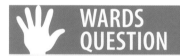

WARDS QUESTION

Q: What is the treatment for Wernicke's encephalopathy?

A: High dose *parenteral* (IV or IM) thiamine should be given for 2–7 days, followed by daily oral thiamine.

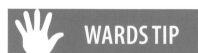

WARDS TIP

Give all patients with altered mental status thiamine *before* glucose, to avoid precipitating Wernicke–Korsakoff syndrome. Thiamine is a coenzyme used in carbohydrate metabolism.

- Acute and can be reversed with thiamine therapy.
- Features: Ataxia (broad-based), confusion, ocular abnormalities (nystagmus, gaze palsies).

■ If left untreated, Wernicke's encephalopathy may progress to **Korsakoff syndrome:**

- Chronic amnestic syndrome.
- Reversible in only about 20% of patients.
- Features: Impaired recent memory, anterograde amnesia, compensatory confabulation (unconsciously making up answers when memory has failed).

Cocaine

Cocaine blocks the reuptake of dopamine, epinephrine, and norepinephrine from the synaptic cleft, causing a stimulant effect. Dopamine plays a role in the behavioral reinforcement ("reward") system of the brain.

INTOXICATION

■ *General:* Euphoria, heightened self-esteem, increase or decrease in blood pressure, tachycardia or bradycardia, nausea, dilated pupils, weight loss, psychomotor agitation or depression, chills, and sweating.

■ *Dangerous:* Seizures, cardiac arrhythmias, hyperthermia, paranoia, and hallucinations (especially tactile). Since cocaine is an indirect sympathomimetic, intoxication mimics the fight-or-flight response.

■ *Deadly:* Cocaine's vasoconstrictive effect may result in myocardial infarction (MI), intracranial hemorrhage, or stroke.

Management

- For mild-to-moderate agitation and anxiety: Reassurance of the patient and benzodiazepines.
- For severe agitation or psychosis: Antipsychotics (e.g., haloperidol).
- Symptomatic support (i.e., control hypertension, arrhythmias).
- Temperature of >102°F should be treated aggressively with an ice bath, cooling blanket, and other supportive measures.

COCAINE USE DISORDER

Treatment of cocaine use disorder:

- There is no Food and Drug Administration (FDA)-approved pharmacotherapy for cocaine use disorder.
- Off-label medications are sometimes used (naltrexone, modafinil, topiramate).
- Psychological interventions (contingency management, relapse prevention, NA, etc.) are the mainstay of treatment.

WITHDRAWAL

- Abrupt abstinence is not life threatening.
- Produces post-intoxication depression ("crash"): Malaise, fatigue, hypersomnolence, depression, anhedonia, hunger, constricted pupils, vivid dreams, psychomotor agitation, or retardation. Occasionally, these patients can become suicidal.
- With mild-to-moderate cocaine use, withdrawal symptoms resolve within 72 hours; with heavy, chronic use, they may last for 1–2 weeks.
- Treatment is supportive, but severe psychiatric symptoms may warrant hospitalization.

Amphetamines

- Classic amphetamines:
  - Block reuptake and facilitate release of dopamine and norepinephrine from nerve endings, causing a stimulant effect.
  - *Examples:* Dextroamphetamine (Dexedrine), methylphenidate (Ritalin), methamphetamine (Desoxyn, "ice," "speed," "crystal meth," "crank").
  - Methamphetamines are easily manufactured in home laboratories using over-the-counter medications (e.g., pseudoephedrine).
  - Methamphetamines are used medically in the treatment of narcolepsy, attention deficit/hyperactivity disorder (ADHD), binge eating, and occasionally depressive disorders.
- Substituted ("designer," "club drugs") amphetamines:
  - Release dopamine, norepinephrine, and serotonin from nerve endings.
  - *Examples:* MDMA ("ecstasy"), MDEA ("eve").
  - Often used in dance clubs and raves.
  - Have both stimulant and hallucinogenic properties.
  - Serotonin syndrome is possible if designer amphetamines are combined with selective serotonin reuptake inhibitors (SSRIs).

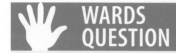

WARDS QUESTION

Q: Why should beta-blockers be avoided for patients who regularly use cocaine?
A: Cocaine has both alpha- and beta-adrenergic effects. If a beta-blocker is given simultaneously, unopposed alpha-adrenergic activity can cause coronary vasoconstriction and induce myocardial infarction.

KEY FACT

Cocaine or amphetamines can both cause *formication*, a tactile hallucination of something crawling on or under the skin.

KEY FACT

Symptoms of amphetamine intoxication include euphoria, dilated pupils, increased libido, tachycardia, perspiration, grinding teeth, and chest pain.

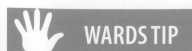

WARDS TIP

Chronic amphetamine use leads to accelerated tooth decay ("meth mouth").

WARDS TIP

Both amphetamine and PCP use can cause rhabdomyolysis. Look for elevated creatine kinase (CK) and monitor closely for acute kidney injury. Treatment is mostly supportive and emphasizes hydration.

KEY FACT

Ketamine ("special K") can produce tachycardia, tachypnea, hallucinations, and amnesia.

KEY FACT

PCP intoxication symptoms—
RED DANES
Rage
Erythema (redness of skin)
Dilated pupils
Delusions
Amnesia
Nystagmus
Excitation
Skin dryness

KEY FACT

Nystagmus (especially rotary) is very common in PCP intoxication.

INTOXICATION

Clinical Presentation

- Amphetamine intoxication causes symptoms similar to those of cocaine (see above).
- MDMA and MDEA may induce sense of closeness to others.
- Overdose can cause hyperthermia, dehydration (especially after a prolonged period of dancing in a club), rhabdomyolysis, and renal failure.
- Complications of their long half-life can cause ongoing psychosis, even during abstinence.
- Amphetamine withdrawal can cause prolonged depression.

Treatment
Rehydrate, correct electrolyte balance, and treat hyperthermia.

Phencyclidine (PCP)

PCP, or "angel dust," is a dissociative, hallucinogenic drug that antagonizes *N*-methyl-D-aspartate (NMDA) glutamate receptors and activates dopaminergic neurons. It can have stimulant or CNS depressant effects, depending on the dose taken.

- PCP can be smoked as "wet" (sprinkled on cigarette) or as a "joint" (sprinkled on marijuana).
- Ketamine is similar to PCP, but is less potent. Ketamine is sometimes used as a "date rape" drug, as it is odorless and tasteless.

INTOXICATION

Clinical Presentation

- Effects include agitation, depersonalization, hallucinations, synesthesia (one sensory stimulation evokes another—e.g., hearing a sound causes one to see a color), impaired judgment, memory impairment, combativeness, **nystagmus** (rotary, horizontal, or vertical), ataxia, dysarthria, hypertension, tachycardia, muscle rigidity, and high tolerance to pain.
- Overdose can cause seizures, delirium, coma, and even death.

Treatment

- Monitor vitals, temperature, and electrolytes, and minimize sensory stimulation.
- Use benzodiazepines (lorazepam) to treat agitation, anxiety, muscle spasms, and seizures.
- Use antipsychotics (haloperidol) to control severe agitation or psychotic symptoms.

WITHDRAWAL

No withdrawal syndrome, but "flashbacks" (recurrence of intoxication symptoms due to release of the drug from body lipid stores) may occur.

Sedative-Hypnotics

Agents in the sedative-hypnotics category include benzodiazepines, barbiturates, zolpidem, zaleplon, gamma-hydroxybutyrate (GHB), meprobamate, and others. These medications, especially benzodiazepines, are highly abused in the United States, as they are more readily available than other drugs such as cocaine.

- Benzodiazepines (BZDs):
  - Commonly used in the treatment of anxiety disorders.
  - Easily obtained via prescription from physicians' offices and emergency departments.
  - Potentiate the effects of GABA by modulating the receptor, thereby increasing frequency of chloride channel opening.
- Barbiturates:
  - Used in the treatment of epilepsy and as anesthetics.
  - Potentiate the effects of GABA by binding to the receptor and increasing duration of chloride channel opening.
  - At high doses, barbiturates act as direct GABA agonists, and therefore have a lower margin of safety relative to BZDs. Overdose can be lethal.
  - They are synergistic in combination with BZDs (as well as other CNS depressants such as alcohol); respiratory depression can occur.

INTOXICATION

Clinical Presentation

- Intoxication with sedatives produces drowsiness, confusion, hypotension, slurred speech, incoordination, ataxia, mood lability, impaired judgment, nystagmus, respiratory depression, and coma or death in overdose.
- Symptoms are synergistic when combined with EtOH or opioids/narcotics.
- Long-term sedative use may lead to dependence and may cause depressive symptoms.

Treatment

- Maintain airway, breathing, and circulation. Monitor vital signs.
- Activated charcoal and gastric lavage to prevent further gastrointestinal absorption (if drug was ingested in the prior 4–6 hours).
- For *barbiturates only:* Alkalinize urine with sodium bicarbonate to promote renal excretion.
- For *benzodiazepines only:* Flumazenil in overdose.
- Supportive care—Improve respiratory status, control hypotension.

WITHDRAWAL

Abrupt abstinence after chronic use can be ***life threatening***. While physiological dependence is more likely with short-acting agents, longer-acting agents can also cause dependence and withdrawal symptoms.

CLINICAL PRESENTATION

Signs and symptoms of withdrawal are the same as these of EtOH withdrawal. Tonic-clonic seizures may occur and can be life threatening.

KEY FACT

PCP intoxication is associated with violence, more so than other drugs.

KEY FACT

Gamma-hydroxybutyrate (GHB) is a CNS depressant that produces confusion, dizziness, drowsiness, memory loss, respiratory distress, and coma. It is commonly used as a date-rape drug.

WARDS QUESTION

Q: Which substances of abuse have potentially fatal withdrawal syndromes?
A: Alcohol, benzodiazepines, and barbiturates.

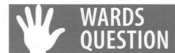

WARDS TIP

Flumazenil is a very short-acting BZD antagonist used for treating BZD overdose. Use with caution when treating overdose, as it may precipitate seizures.

KEY FACT

The opioid dextromethorphan is a common ingredient in cough syrup.

KEY FACT

Infection secondary to needle sharing is a common cause of morbidity from street heroin usage.

KEY FACT

Opioid intoxication: Nausea, vomiting, sedation, decrease in pain perception, decrease in gastrointestinal motility, pupil constriction, and respiratory depression (which *can be fatal*).

KEY FACT

Meperidine is the exception to opioids producing miosis. "Demerol Dilates pupils."

KEY FACT

Naloxone is the treatment of choice for opiate overdose.

WARDS TIP

Classic triad of opioid overdose—**R**ebels **A**dmire **M**orphine
Respiratory depression
Altered mental status
Miosis

Treatment

- Benzodiazepines (stabilize patient, then taper gradually).
- Carbamazepine or valproic acid taper not as beneficial.

Opioids

- Opioid medications and drugs of abuse stimulate mu, kappa, and delta opiate receptors (normally stimulated by endogenous opiates), and are involved in analgesia, sedation, and dependence. Examples include heroin, oxycodone, codeine, dextromethorphan, morphine, methadone, and meperidine (Demerol).
- Opioids also have effects on the dopaminergic system, which mediates their addictive and rewarding properties.
- Prescription opioids (OxyContin [oxycodone], Vicodin [hydrocodone/acetaminophen], and Percocet [oxycodone/acetaminophen])—not heroin—are the most commonly used opioids.
- Behaviors such as losing medication, "doctor shopping," and running out of medication early should alert clinicians of possible misuse.
- Opioids are associated with more deaths (usually due to unintentional overdose) than any other drug.

INTOXICATION

Clinical Presentation

- Opioid intoxication causes drowsiness, nausea/vomiting, constipation, slurred speech, **constricted pupils**, seizures, and respiratory depression, which may progress to coma or death in overdose.
- Meperidine and monoamine oxidase inhibitors taken in combination may cause **serotonin syndrome**: hyperthermia, confusion, hypertension or hypotension, and hyperreflexia.

Treatment

- Ensure adequate airway, breathing, and circulation.
- In overdose, administration of naloxone (an opioid antagonist) will improve respiratory depression but may cause severe withdrawal in an opioid-dependent patient.
- Ventilatory support may be required.
- Patients at risk of opioid overdose should be prescribed a naloxone (Narcan) kit to keep at home for emergencies.

OPIATE USE DISORDER

See Table 7-7 for treatment of opioid use disorder.

WITHDRAWAL

- While not life threatening, abstinence in the opioid-dependent individual leads to an unpleasant withdrawal syndrome characterized by dysphoria, insomnia, lacrimation, rhinorrhea, yawning, weakness, sweating, piloerection, nausea/vomiting, fever, dilated pupils, abdominal cramps, arthralgia/myalgia, hypertension, tachycardia, and craving.

TABLE 7-7. Pharmacological Treatment of Opioid Use Disorder			
Medication	Mechanism	Pros	Cons
Methadone	Full agonist at mu-opioid receptor.	Administered once daily. Long half life.	Restricted to federally licensed substance abuse treatment programs. Can cause QTc interval prolongation: screening electrocardiogram is indicated, particularly in patients with high risk of cardiac disease.
		Presenting to the methadone clinic for regular pickups can be helpful for patients who benefit from daily structure and access to group therapy or case management.	Patients can still use other opioids on top of methadone.
Buprenorphine	Partial opioid receptor agonist—can precipitate withdrawal if used too soon after full opioid agonists.	Sublingual preparation that is safer than methadone, as its effects reach a plateau and make overdose unlikely.	In the outpatient setting, can only be prescribed by a physician with a special waiver on their controlled substances license.
		Combined formulation (buprenorphine-naloxone, or Suboxone) prevents intoxication from intravenous or intranasal use.	
Naltrexone	Competitive opioid antagonist, precipitates withdrawal if used within 7 days of heroin use	Available as daily oral medication or monthly depot injection. It is a good choice for highly motivated patients such as health care professionals.	Adherence is an issue for oral formulation. Risk of LFT elevation. Can interfere with anesthesia (e.g., for acute injuries or surgical procedures).
Naloxone	Competitive opioid antagonist, used in treatment of overdose.	Can be life-saving for patients or their peers, and should routinely be prescribed for all patients with opioid use disorder (especially for those who are receiving medication-assisted treatment).	Does not reduce opioid use or treat symptoms of opioid use disorder.
			Very short half-life; patients must be educated about need to call EMS or present to ED after it's administered (even if the overdose appears to be reversed).

- Treatment includes:
  - Moderate symptoms: Symptomatic treatment with clonidine (for autonomic signs and symptoms of withdrawal), nonsteroidal anti-inflammatory drugs (NSAIDs) for pain, loperamide for diarrhea, dicyclomine for abdominal cramps, promethazine for nausea, etc.
  - Severe symptoms: Detox with buprenorphine or methadone.
  - Monitor degree of withdrawal with COWS (Clinical Opioid Withdrawal Scale), which uses objective measures (i.e., pulse, pupil size, tremor) to assess withdrawal severity.

 KEY FACT

Eating large amounts of poppy seed bagels or muffins can result in a urine drug screen that is positive for opioids.

Hallucinogens

Hallucinogenic drugs of abuse include psilocybin (mushrooms), mescaline (peyote cactus), and lysergic acid diethylamide (LSD). Pharmacological effects vary, but LSD is believed to act on the serotonergic system. Hallucinogens do not cause physical dependence or withdrawal, though users can rarely develop psychological dependence.

INTOXICATION

- Effects include perceptual changes (illusions, hallucinations, body image distortions, synesthesia), labile affect, dilated pupils, tachycardia, hypertension, hyperthermia, tremors, incoordination, sweating, and palpitations.

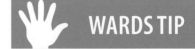 **WARDS TIP**

Rapid recovery of consciousness following the administration of intravenous (IV) naloxone (a potent opioid antagonist) is consistent with opioid overdose.

KEY FACT

Remember the withdrawal symptoms of opiates: flu-like symptoms (body aches, anorexia, rhinorrhea, fever), diarrhea, anxiety, insomnia, and piloerection. These are **not** life threatening.

KEY FACT

An LSD flashback is a spontaneous recurrence of symptoms mimicking a prior LSD "trip" that may last for minutes to hours.

KEY FACT

Dronabinol is a pill form of THC that is FDA-approved for certain indications.

- Usually lasts 6–12 hours, but may last for several days.
- May have a "bad trip" that consists of marked anxiety, panic, and psychotic symptoms (paranoia, hallucinations).
- **Treatment**: Monitor for dangerous behavior and reassure patient. Use benzodiazepines as first-line for agitation (can use antipsychotics if needed).

WITHDRAWAL

No withdrawal syndrome is produced, but with long-term LSD use, patients may experience flashbacks later in life.

Marijuana

- Cannabis ("marijuana," "pot," "weed," "grass") is the most commonly used illicit substance in the world.
- The main psychoactive component which produces the "high" in cannabis is THC (tetrahydrocannabinol).
- Cannabinoid receptors in the brain inhibit adenylate cyclase.
- Marijuana has shown some efficacy in treating nausea and vomiting in chemotherapy patients, increasing appetite in AIDS patients, in chronic pain (from cancer), and lowering intraocular pressure in glaucoma. A specific class of compounds found in marijuana, cannabidiols (CBDs), is currently being studied for management of pain, seizures, and anxiety/depression.

INTOXICATION

- Marijuana causes euphoria, anxiety, impaired motor coordination, perceptual disturbances (sensation of slowed time), mild tachycardia, anxiety, conjunctival injection (red eyes), dry mouth, and increased appetite ("the munchies").
- Cannabis-induced psychotic disorders with paranoia, hallucinations, and/or delusions may occur. There is no overdose syndrome for marijuana use.
- Cannabis use disorder occurs in approximately 10% of those who use (up to 50% of daily users).
- Chronic use may cause respiratory problems such as asthma and chronic bronchitis, immunosuppression, cancer, and possible effects on reproductive hormones.
- **Treatment**: Supportive, psychosocial interventions (e.g., contingency management, groups).

WITHDRAWAL

- Withdrawal symptoms may include irritability, anxiety, restlessness, aggression, strange dreams, depression, headaches, sweating, chills, insomnia, and low appetite.
- **Treatment**: Supportive and symptomatic.

Inhalants

- Inhalants include a broad range of drugs that are inhaled and absorbed through the lungs.

- Inhalants generally act as CNS depressants.
- Most commonly used by preadolescents or adolescents; rate of use is similar between boys and girls (but rare in adult females).
- *Examples:* Solvents, glue, paint thinners, fuels, isobutyl nitrates ("huffing," "laughing gas," "rush," "bolt").

INTOXICATION

- **Effects:** Perceptual disturbances, paranoia, lethargy, dizziness, nausea/vomiting, headache, nystagmus, tremor, muscle weakness, hyporeflexia, ataxia, slurred speech, euphoria, hypoxia, clouding of consciousness, stupor, or coma.
- Acute intoxication: 15–30 minutes. May be sustained with repeated use.
- **Overdose:** May be fatal secondary to respiratory depression or cardiac arrhythmias.
- Long-term use may cause permanent damage to CNS (e.g., neurocognitive impairment, cerebellar dysfunction, Parkinsonism, seizures), peripheral neuropathy, myopathy, aplastic anemia, malignancy, metabolic acidosis, urinary calculi, glomerulonephritis, myocarditis, MI, and hepatotoxicity.
- **Treatment:** Monitor airway, breathing, and circulation; may need oxygen with hypoxic states.
- Identify solvent because some (e.g., leaded gasoline) may require chelation.

WITHDRAWAL

A withdrawal syndrome does not usually occur, but symptoms may include irritability, sleep disturbance, anxiety, depression, nausea, vomiting, and craving.

Caffeine

Caffeine is the most commonly used psychoactive substance in the United States, usually in the form of coffee, tea, or energy drinks. It acts as an adenosine antagonist, causing increase in cyclic adenosine monophosphate (cAMP) and stimulating the release of excitatory neurotransmitters.

OVERDOSE

- More than 250 mg (2 cups of coffee): Anxiety, insomnia, muscle twitching, rambling speech, flushed face, diuresis, gastrointestinal disturbance, restlessness, excitement, and tachycardia.
- More than 1 g: May cause tinnitus, severe agitation, visual light flashes, and cardiac arrhythmias.
- More than 10 g: Death may occur secondary to seizures and respiratory failure.
- **Treatment:** Supportive and symptomatic.

WITHDRAWAL

- Caffeine withdrawal symptoms occur in 50–75% of caffeine users if cessation is abrupt.
- Withdrawal symptoms include **headache**, fatigue, irritability, nausea, vomiting, drowsiness, muscle pain, and depression.
- Usually resolves within 1½ weeks.

WARDS TIP

Cigarette smoking during pregnancy is associated with low birth weight, SIDS, and a variety of postnatal morbidities.

Nicotine

- Nicotine is derived from the tobacco plant, and stimulates nicotinic receptors in autonomic ganglia of the sympathetic and parasympathetic nervous systems. It is highly addictive through its effects on the dopaminergic system.
- Nicotine use causes both tolerance and physical dependence (i.e., prominent craving and withdrawal).
- Cigarette smoking is the leading cause of preventable morbidity and mortality in the United States, posing many health risks including chronic obstructive pulmonary disease (COPD), cardiovascular diseases, and various cancers.
- Current smoking prevalence is about 15% of U.S. adults.
- Effects: Restlessness, insomnia, anxiety, and increase in gastrointestinal motility.
- **Withdrawal symptoms**: Intense craving, dysphoria, anxiety, poor concentration, increase in appetite, weight gain, irritability, restlessness, and insomnia.

TREATMENT OF NICOTINE DEPENDENCE

FDA-approved pharmacotherapy:

- Varenicline (Chantix): $\alpha4\beta2$ nicotinic cholinergic receptor (nAChR) partial agonist that mimics the action of nicotine, reducing the rewarding aspects and preventing withdrawal symptoms.
- Bupropion (Zyban): Antidepressant inhibits reuptake of dopamine and norepinephrine; helps reduce craving and withdrawal symptoms.
- Nicotine replacement therapy (NRT): Available as transdermal patch, gum, lozenge, nasal spray, and inhaler.
- Behavioral support/counseling should be part of every treatment.
- Relapse after abstinence is common.

Gambling Disorder

DIAGNOSIS AND *DSM-5* CRITERIA

Persistent and recurrent problematic gambling behavior, as evidenced by four or more of the following in a 12-month period:

1. Preoccupation with gambling.
2. Need to gamble with increasing amount of money to achieve pleasure.
3. Repeated and unsuccessful attempts to cut down on or stop gambling.
4. Restlessness or irritability when attempting to stop gambling.
5. Gambling when feeling distressed (depressed, anxious, etc.).
6. Returning to reclaim losses after gambling ("get even").
7. Lying to hide level of gambling.
8. Jeopardizing relationships or job because of gambling.
9. Relying on others to financially support gambling.

EPIDEMIOLOGY/ETIOLOGY

- Prevalence: 0.4–1.0% of adults in the United States.
- Men represent most of the cases.
- More common in young adults and middle-aged, and lower rates in older adults.
- Similar to substance use disorders, the course is marked by periods of abstinence and relapse.
- Increased incidence of mood disorders, anxiety disorders, substance use disorders, and personality disorders.
- Etiology may involve genetic, temperamental, environmental, and neurochemical factors.
- One-third may achieve recovery without treatment.

TREATMENT

- Participation in Gamblers Anonymous (a 12-step program) is the most common treatment.
- Cognitive-behavioral therapy has been shown to be effective, particularly when combined with Gamblers Anonymous.
- Important to treat comorbid mood disorders, anxiety disorders, and substance use disorders where appropriate.

NOTES

Definition

The neurocognitive disorders (NCDs) comprise a group of conditions defined by decline from a previous level of cognitive functioning. The six cognitive domains that may be affected include **complex attention**, **executive function**, **learning and memory**, **language**, **perceptual-motor skills**, and **social cognition (interaction)**. By definition, cause(s) for the deficits may be ascertained from findings on history, physical exam, and diagnostic testing. The *DSM-5* divides the NCDs into three main categories: delirium, mild NCDs, and major NCDs (dementias).

Delirium

- Delirium is a **medical emergency**.
- May be the only early manifestation of serious illness.
- Potentially reversible.
- Can advance to coma, seizures, or death.
- Associated with **high mortality**. Up to 40% of individuals die within 1 year of diagnosis.

EPIDEMIOLOGY

- Up to one-half of hospitalized elderly patients develop delirium.
- As many as 90% of patients with a preexisting NCD (dementia) will experience a superimposed delirium when admitted to the hospital.
- Delirium often goes unrecognized (65–88% of the time).
- Delirium is associated with an increased risk for later development of major NCD.

RISK FACTORS

- Advanced age.
- Preexisting cognitive impairment or depression.
- Prior history of delirium.
- Severe or terminal illness.
- Multiple medical comorbidities.
- Hearing or vision impairment.

PRECIPITATING FACTORS

- Polypharmacy, including the use of psychotropic medications (especially benzodiazepines and anticholinergic drugs).
- Alcohol use or withdrawal.
- Infection.
- Pain.
- Dehydration.
- Malnutrition.
- Impaired mobility.
- Sleep deprivation.
- Organ failure.
- Mechanical ventilation.

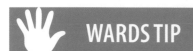

WARDS TIP

Terms commonly used for delirium include *toxic* or *metabolic encephalopathy, acute organic brain syndrome, acute confusional state, acute toxic psychosis*, and *ICU psychosis*.

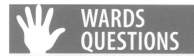

WARDS TIP

Consider delirium as acute brain failure—a *medical emergency* like other acute organ failures.

WARDS QUESTIONS

Q: What is the "ICU triad?"
A: **P**ain, **A**gitation, and **D**elirium.

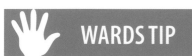

WARDS TIP

Delirium is commonly experienced by patients in the ICU and postoperative recovery.

TABLE 8-1. Clinical Scenarios of Delirium on Exam		
Scenario	Likely Diagnosis	Diagnostic Testing
Delirium + fever + cough + rales	Pneumonia	Chest x-ray
Delirium + dysuria + suprapubic tenderness	Urinary tract infection	Urinalysis and urine culture
Delirium + constricted pupils (miosis) + bradypnea	Opioid intoxication	Urine toxicology screen
Delirium + fever + nuchal rigidity + photophobia	Meningitis	Lumbar puncture
Delirium + tachycardia + tremor + thyromegaly	Thyrotoxicosis	TSH, free T_4, T_3
Delirium + insulin use	Hypoglycemia	Blood glucose

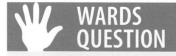

WARDS TIP

Common causes of medication-induced delirium:

- Anticholinergics
- Benzodiazepines
- Nonbenzodiazepine hypnotics ("Z-drugs")
- Opioids (especially meperidine)
- Corticosteroids
- Tricyclic antidepressants
- H2 blockers

ETIOLOGY

- Almost any medical condition can cause delirium (see examples in Table 8-1).
- The *DSM-5* recognizes five broad categories:
  - Substance intoxication delirium.
  - Substance withdrawal delirium.
  - Medication-induced delirium.
  - Delirium due to another medical condition.
  - Delirium due to multiple etiologies.

CLINICAL MANIFESTATIONS

- Primarily a disorder of **attention** and **awareness** (i.e., **orientation**).
- Cognitive deficits **develop acutely** over hours to days.
- Symptoms **fluctuate** throughout the course of a day, typically worsening at night.
- Other features include deficits in **recent memory**, language abnormalities, or perceptual disturbances (usually **visual**, such as illusions or hallucinations).
- Circadian rhythm disruption and emotional symptoms are common.
- There are three types of delirium based on psychomotor activity.
  - Purely hypoactive ("quiet") type
    - Decreased psychomotor activity, ranging from drowsiness to lethargy to stupor.
    - **More likely to go undetected.**
    - More common in the elderly.
  - Purely hyperactive type ("ICU psychosis")
    - Manifests with agitation, mood lability, and uncooperativeness.
    - More easily identified due to its disruptiveness.
    - More common in **drug withdrawal or toxicity**.
  - Mixed type
    - Psychomotor activity may remain stable at baseline or fluctuate rapidly between hyperactivity and hypoactivity.
- Hospitalized patients usually recover within 1 week, although some degree of cognitive deficits can persist for months or even indefinitely.

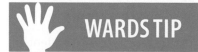

WARDS QUESTION

Q: What are the two most common precipitants of delirium in children?
A: Febrile illnesses and medications.

WARDS TIP

Suspect delirium if a patient presents with altered mental status, disorientation, confusion, agitation, or sudden onset of psychotic symptoms.

WARDS TIP

A quick, first-glance bedside exam for suspected substance/medication intoxication is **VALEUMS**.

- **V**ital signs
- **A**lertness **L**evel
- **E**yes (pupil size and position)
- **U**rine (bladder distention or incontinence)
- **M**ucous membranes (moisture)
- **S**kin (temperature and moisture)

KEY FACT

Delirium generally manifests as diffuse background slowing on electroencephalography (EEG). An exception is delirium tremens, which is associated with fast EEG activity. EEG lacks sensitivity and specificity for making the diagnosis but is useful for ruling out nonconvulsive seizures.

WARDS TIP

Consider obtaining a head CT for a patient with delirium under the following circumstances:

- No underlying cause evident on initial evaluation.
- In the context of head trauma.
- New focal neurologic deficits detected on exam.
- Patient is unable or unwilling to cooperate with a neurologic examination.
- No improvement despite treatment of already identified causes.

TABLE 8-2. *DSM-5* Criteria for Delirium
■ Disturbance in **attention** and **awareness**.
■ Disturbance in **an additional cognitive domain**.
■ Develops **acutely** over hours to days, represents a **change** from baseline, and tends to **fluctuate**.
■ **Not** better accounted for by **another neurocognitive disorder**.
■ **Not** occurring during a **coma**.
■ Evidence from history, physical, or labs that the disturbance is a **direct consequence** of **another medical condition**, **substance intoxication/withdrawal**, exposure to **toxin**, or due to multiple etiologies.

DIAGNOSIS

- Table 8-2 summarizes the *DSM-5* diagnostic criteria.
- A useful clinical tool for evaluation of a patient with suspected delirium is the **Confusion Assessment Method** (CAM).
  - This method takes 5 minutes to perform and has a high sensitivity and specificity.
  - Delirium is diagnosed in a patient with **inattention** of **acute onset** and/or **fluctuating course** along with either **disorganized thinking** or **altered consciousness**.
    - Inattention manifests as distractibility or difficulty maintaining focus during the evaluation.
    - Disorganized thinking is demonstrated via derailment or loose associations.
    - Level of consciousness ranges from vigilant (hyperalert) to alert (normal) to lethargic (drowsy, but easily aroused) to stuporous (difficult to arouse) to comatose (unarousable to verbal stimulation).
- Once delirium has been diagnosed, the cause(s) should be sought.
  - Finger-stick blood glucose, pulse-oximetry, arterial blood gases, and electrocardiography can quickly provide useful data at bedside.
  - Labs typically obtained in a delirium workup include a basic metabolic panel, serum magnesium, complete blood count with differential, urinalysis, and urine culture.
  - Urine and blood drug screen, blood alcohol level, therapeutic drug levels (e.g., antiepileptics, digoxin, lithium), hepatic panel, thyroid hormone levels, inflammatory markers (e.g., C-reactive protein, erythrocyte sedimentation rate), vitamin B12 level, or chest x-ray may also be warranted depending on the clinical presentation.
  - Head imaging (head CT or brain MRI), EEG, and lumbar puncture should be performed if focal neurological deficits are present or a cause of delirium cannot be identified with the initial workup.

TREATMENT

- **Treat the underlying cause(s)**.
- Address potential exacerbating factors: Mobility limitations, sensory deficits, sleep cycle disruption, constipation, urinary retention, dehydration, electrolyte abnormalities, uncontrolled pain, and medications.

- Encourage a family member to stay at the bedside to help with supervision and orientation.

- Utilize a one-to-one sitter if needed.

- Reorient the patient on a regular basis regarding time, place, and situation. Open window shades during the day and place whiteboards, calendars, and clocks in plain sight.

- D2 antagonists (i.e., antipsychotics) are indicated for treatment of agitation that endangers the patient or others.

  - **Haloperidol** is the preferred agent and can be administered orally, intramuscularly, or intravenously.

  - D2 antagonists exacerbate extrapyramidal symptoms; use with caution in patients with Parkinsonism.

- Avoid benzodiazepines (except in alcohol or benzodiazepine withdrawal) as they may worsen the delirium by causing paradoxical disinhibition or over-sedation.

- Avoid the use of restraints. They can worsen agitation and cause injury. When restraints are necessary, reassess often and remove as soon as possible. Use the least restrictive means appropriate for the situation.

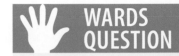

WARDS QUESTION

Q: In what scenarios is it appropriate to use benzodiazepines to treat delirium?
A: Alcohol and benzodiazepine withdrawal.

 An 83-year-old female is admitted to the hospital after presenting with a fever and altered mental status. Her home nurse aide reports that the patient was in her usual state of health until 24 hours prior to admission when she became confused and seemed to be talking to herself. In a few hours, her mental status improved then deteriorated again. After the patient dialed 911 to report that she was being held hostage by terrorists, her nurse aid called an ambulance on her behalf.

On examination, the patient is somnolent and has difficulty responding to questions appropriately. She is disoriented to place and time.

When the daughter calls to check in, she shares that her mother has had progressive memory deficits over the past several years. The patient can no longer drive and requires assistance with finances and meal preparation.

What is the most likely acute diagnosis?

The patient most likely has delirium. She presents with a sudden change in cognition as manifested by confusion, disorientation, and hallucinations. She has had an acute change from her baseline behavior. Her symptoms wax and wane throughout the day, representing the typical fluctuation found in delirium. She presents with a fever, likely secondary to an infection. If confirmed, her diagnosis would be delirium due to the specific infectious etiology.

Collateral information points to a prior diagnosis of major neurocognitive disorder (dementia). She has a history of memory impairment that began gradually and has progressively worsened. There is also history of impairment in executive functioning, and she can no longer care for herself. The existence of a major neurocognitive disorder is a risk factor for the development of a superimposed delirium.

Mild and Major Neurocognitive Disorders

■ The non-delirium NCDs are characterized by a chronic cognitive decline that impacts functioning in daily activities (Table 8-3).

■ Individuals with **mild NCDs** (mild cognitive impairment [MCI] or cognitive impairment, no dementia [CIND]) experience difficulty with some of the more complex activities of daily living but are able to maintain their independence.

■ Patients with **major NCDs** require assistance with independent activities of daily living (IADLs), such as paying bills, managing medications, or shopping for groceries. Over time, the basic activities of daily living (e.g., feeding, toileting, bathing) are affected, eventually leading to total dependence.

■ The mild and major NCDs are also subcategorized by etiology (Table 8-4).

• The **dementias** comprise a large group of progressive and irreversible major NCDs that primarily affect the elderly.

• Several other major NCDs present similarly to the dementias, but their progression may be arrested or even reversed with treatment (e.g., vitamin B12 deficiency, thyroid dysfunction, normal pressure hydrocephalus).

DIAGNOSIS

■ The **Mini Mental State Exam (MMSE)** is a screening test used due to its speed and ease of administration.

• Assesses orientation, attention/concentration, language, constructional ability, and immediate and delayed recall.

• Sensitive for major NCDs (e.g., dementias), particularly moderate-to-severe forms.

  - Perfect score: 30.

  - Dysfunction: <25.

• Not as sensitive for mild NCDs and early major NCDs.

• Lacks specificity.

• Norm tables are available to adjust for age and education.

KEY FACT

Thyroid dysfunction can cause reversible cognitive impairment. Hypothyroidism is typically accompanied by fatigue and cold intolerance. Hyperthyroidism in the elderly may manifest as an "apathetic thyrotoxicosis," characterized by depression and lethargy. Thyroid function tests are often included in the initial workup of any new onset psychiatric illness.

TABLE 8-3. *DSM-5* Criteria for Mild and Major NCDs		
Criterion	Mild NCDs	Major NCDs
Functional decline in at least one cognitive domain relative to baseline as evidenced by		
Concern (expressed by the patient or caretaker)	Mild decline	Significant decline
Objective findings on cognitive testing (preferably standardized neuropsychological testing)	Modest impairment	Substantial impairment
Effect on functioning in daily life.	Ability to perform IADLs preserved	Impaired performance of IADLs/ADLs
Deficits do not occur exclusively in the context of a delirium		
Deficits are not better explained by another mental disorder.		

ADLs, basic activities of daily living; IADLs, independent activities of daily living.

TABLE 8-4. Clinical Scenarios of Neurocognitive Disorders on Exam	
Scenario	**Likely Diagnosis**
>65-year-old patient with memory impairment + executive dysfunction + poor insight progressing later to psychiatric/behavioral disturbances + insomnia + apraxia.	Alzheimer disease
>65-year-old patient with executive dysfunction + cognitive slowing + **stepwise** progression ± focal neurologic abnormalities ± history of known **stroke**.	Vascular NCD
>60-year-old patient with **gait apraxia** + **urinary urgency** → **incontinence** + executive dysfunction + apathy.	Normal pressure hydrocephalus
>50-year-old patient with **parkinsonism preceding cognitive decline** by several years.	Parkinson disease
>50-year-old patient with **concomitant development** of cognitive impairment (**visuospatial dysfunction**) + parkinsonism, as well as **REM sleep behaviors** + fluctuating alertness level + visual hallucinations.	NCD with Lewy bodies
Patient of any age with cognitive slowing + short-term memory impairment + **fatigue** + **cold intolerance**.	Hypothyroidism
Patient of any age with cognitive slowing + depression + **vegan diet** + paresthesias/numbness + ataxia.	Vitamin B12 deficiency

- Another commonly used screening tool is the **Mini-Cog**.
  - Consists of three-item recall and clock-drawing tasks.
  - Positive screening for cognitive impairment:
    - No items recalled after 3 minutes.
    - Only one to two items recalled with abnormal clock drawing.
  - Negative screening:
    - All three items repeated correctly after 3 minutes.
    - One to two items recalled with normal clock drawing.
- Other commonly used screening tools include:
  - Blessed Orientation-Memory-Concentration (BOMC).
  - Montreal Cognitive Assessment (MoCA).
  - Frontal Assessment Battery (FAB).
- An abnormal screening test indicates the need for further testing, preferably formal neuropsychological testing.

ALZHEIMER DISEASE (AD)

Alzheimer disease is the **most common** underlying etiology of major NCDs (dementias).

Clinical Manifestations
- **Gradually progressive decline** in cognitive functions.
- The primary cognitive domains affected are **memory**, **learning**, and **language**.
- Personality changes, mood swings, and paranoia are very common.
- Motor and sensory symptoms appear in advanced disease.
- Death often occurs within 10 years of diagnosis.

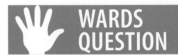

WARDS QUESTION

Q: What are the "four As" of Alzheimer disease?
A: **A**mnesia, **a**gnosia, **a**praxia, and **a**phasia.

KEY FACT

Postmortem pathological examination of the brain is the only way to definitively diagnose Alzheimer disease.

KEY FACT

Senile plaques and neurofibrillary tangles are found in Alzheimer disease, as well as Down syndrome and even in normal aging.

KEY FACT

Adults with Down syndrome are at increased risk of developing Alzheimer disease in midlife.

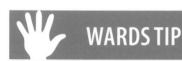

WARDS TIP

Antipsychotics carry a black box warning about increased risk of death in patients with dementia.

Diagnosis

- A diagnosis of **possible** NCD due to AD is made based on the presence of characteristic clinical findings:
  - Insidious onset.
  - Gradual progression.
  - Impairment in one (mild NCD) or more (major NCD) cognitive domains.
- NCD due to AD is **probable** if there is evidence of causation by one of several single-gene variants.

Etiology

- Accumulation of extraneuronal *beta*-amyloid plaques and intraneuronal *tau* protein tangles is associated with progressive brain atrophy.
- Approximately 1% of AD results from an autosomal dominant single-gene mutation (amyloid precursor protein, presenilin 1, or presenilin 2), which is associated with an early onset of symptoms.
- The *epsilon*-4 variant of the *apolipoprotein* gene is a risk factor for developing early-onset AD.

Epidemiology

- AD pathology is estimated to play a role in 60–90% of major NCDs.
- Approximately 50% of patients with AD pathology have an NCD due to multiple etiologies.
- Two-thirds of patients diagnosed with AD are female.
- Diagnosis is made after the age of 65 in the vast majority of individuals.

Treatment

- No cure or truly effective treatment yet available.
- **Cholinesterase inhibitors** (e.g., donepezil, rivastigmine, and galantamine) may slow clinical deterioration by 6–12 months in up to 50% of patients with mild-to-moderate AD.
- The **NMDA receptor antagonist**, memantine, may provide a modest benefit to patients with moderate-to-severe disease.
- Antipsychotic medications are often used to treat agitation and aggression.
  - Because they are associated with **increased mortality** in patients with dementia, low doses should be prescribed for short periods of time.
  - Ideally, informed consent should be obtained from patients and/or their designated decision makers.
  - **Monitor closely** for side effects.
- Supportive care via behavioral, social, and environmental interventions.
- A **multidisciplinary approach** is necessary.
- Any treatment plan must include **caregiver support**.

VASCULAR DISEASE (VASCULAR COGNITIVE IMPAIRMENT)

- Second most common single cause of major NCD.
- Evidence of vascular disease is found in half of all major NCDs, most commonly comorbid with AD pathology (NCD due to multiple etiologies).

- Cognitive decline occurs as a result of at least one of the following mechanisms:
  - Large vessel strokes, usually cortical.
  - Small vessel strokes (lacunar infarcts) to subcortical structures.
  - Microvascular disease affecting the periventricular white matter.
- Effects vary based on the size, location, and number of infarcts.

Risk Factors

- Hypertension.
- Diabetes.
- Smoking.
- Obesity.
- Hyperlipidemia.
- Atrial fibrillation.
- Coronary artery disease.
- Advanced age.

Clinical Manifestations

- Presentation and progression of cognitive impairment are variable.
  - Classically demonstrates a stepwise deterioration corresponding with the occurrence of micro-infarcts (i.e., multi-infarct dementia).
  - May present with acute onset followed by partial improvement.
  - May have an insidious onset with gradual decline similar to AD.
- **Complex attention** and **executive function** are the cognitive domains typically affected in small vessel disease.
- Confirmation of the diagnosis requires neuroimaging with clinical correlation.

Treatment

- No cure or truly effective treatment yet available.
- Manage and mitigate risk factors with the goal of preventing future strokes.
- Symptomatic treatment is similar to AD.

> **KEY FACT**
>
> A lesion to the frontal lobe can manifest with a spectrum of symptoms including personality changes, disinhibition, inappropriate behavior, aggression, apathy, amotivation, and paranoia.

A 68-year-old female is brought to the clinic by her husband. He reports that his wife has recently seemed confused and overly emotional. The patient is able to complete her daily activities, but reports increased difficulty with planning and decision-making. Her medical history is significant for hypertension and transient ischemic attacks (TIAs). A physical exam reveals a carotid bruit.

What is the likely diagnosis?

Mild vascular NCD.

LEWY BODY DISEASE (LBD)

As reflected in its name, the major pathologic features of LBD are Lewy bodies (pathologic aggregations of *alpha*-synuclein) and Lewy neurites in the brain, primarily in the basal ganglia.

Clinical Manifestations

- Progressive cognitive decline.
- Commonly coexists with AD and/or cerebrovascular disease as NCD due to multiple etiologies.
- Core features:
  - **Waxing and waning** of cognition, especially in the areas of **attention** and **alertness**.
  - **Visual hallucinations**—Usually vivid, colorful, well-formed images of (commonly small) people, animals, or objects.
  - **Rapid eye movement** (REM) **sleep behavior disorder** (not included in the *DSM-5* core features but often associated)—Violent movements during sleep in response to dreams (often fighting).
  - Development of **extrapyramidal signs** (Parkinsonism) at least 1 year after cognitive decline becomes evident.
- Suggestive features:
  - Pronounced **antipsychotic sensitivity** (i.e., extrapyramidal symptoms).
  - Postural instability and recurrent falls.
  - Loss of consciousness or transient unresponsiveness.
  - Autonomic dysfunction.
  - Olfactory agnosia or diminished sense of smell.
  - Nonvisual hallucinations and delusions.
  - Excessive sleepiness.
  - Depression, apathy, and anxiety.
- Indicative biomarkers:
  - REM sleep without atonia (RWSA) demonstrated via polysomnography.
  - Decreased 123iodine-MIBG uptake on myocardial scintigraphy.
  - Evidence of reduced dopamine receptor uptake in the basal ganglia via SPECT or PET.

Diagnosis

- Definitive diagnosis can only be made with autopsy.
- **Possible** NCD with Lewy bodies: Only one core feature without evidence from indicative biomarkers OR one or more indicative biomarker(s), but no core clinical features.
- **Probable** NCD with Lewy bodies: Two or more core features OR one core feature and one or more indicative biomarker(s).

Treatment

- **Cholinesterase inhibitors** for cognitive and behavioral symptoms.
- **Quetiapine** or **clozapine** for psychotic symptoms.
  - Use the lowest effective dose for the shortest period of time possible.
  - Monitor closely for adverse effects, such as extrapyramidal signs, sedation, increased confusion, autonomic dysfunction, and signs of **neuroleptic malignant syndrome (NMS)**.
- Levodopa-carbidopa for Parkinsonism.
  - Not as effective as in idiopathic Parkinson disease.
  - May exacerbate psychosis or REM sleep behavior disorder.
- Melatonin and/or clonazepam for REM sleep behavior disorder.

FRONTOTEMPORAL DEGENERATION (FTD)

- FTD includes a diverse group of clinical and pathological disorders that typically present between the ages of 45 and 65.
- Approximately 40% are familial, and 10% are autosomal dominant.

Clinical Manifestations

- Cognitive deficits in **attention**, **abstraction**, **planning**, and **problem solving**.
- **Behavioral variant:**
  - **Disinhibited** verbal, physical, or sexual behavior.
  - Overeating or oral exploration of inanimate objects.
  - Lack of emotional warmth, empathy, or sympathy.
  - Apathy or inertia.
  - Perseveration, repetitive speech, rituals, or obsessions.
  - Decline in **social cognition** and/or **executive abilities**.
- **Language variant** (primary progressive aphasia):
  - Difficulties with **speech** and **comprehension**.
- Relative sparing of learning/memory and perceptual-motor function.
- Many individuals have features of both the behavioral and language variants.
- Increased sensitivity to adverse effects of antipsychotics.

Pathology
Marked atrophy of the frontal and temporal lobes.

Diagnosis

- Definitive diagnosis cannot be made until autopsy.
- FTD is **probable** if frontotemporal atrophy is evident on structural imaging or hypoactivity is visualized on functional imaging with clinical correlates.

Treatment

- Symptom-focused.
- Serotonergic medications (e.g., SSRIs, trazodone) may help reduce disinhibition, anxiety, impulsivity, repetitive behaviors, and eating disorders.

HIV INFECTION

- HIV is the most common infectious agent known to cause cognitive impairment.
- In patients with HIV, 33% have asymptomatic neurocognitive impairment that appears on exam, 12% have mild NCD, and 2% have major NCD.
- Severe forms of NCD due to HIV infection have become much less common with the widespread use of antiretroviral drugs.

Risk Factors

- History of severe immunosuppression.
- High viral loads in the CSF.
- Advanced HIV infection.

Clinical Manifestations

- Variable presentation depending on the part(s) of the brain affected.
- Decline may be observed in executive functioning, attention, working memory, and psychomotor activity.
- Psychiatric and neuromotor symptoms may also be present.

Diagnosis

Mild or major NCD attributable to confirmed HIV infection.

Treatment

- Antiretroviral therapy (ART) improves cognition in some patients.
- Psychostimulants target fatigue, apathy, and psychomotor retardation.

HUNTINGTON DISEASE (HD)

- A genetic disorder resulting from trinucleotide (CAG) repeats in the gene encoding the huntingtin (HTT) protein on chromosome 4.
- Autosomal dominant mode of inheritance.

Clinical Manifestations

- Characterized by a triad of **motor**, **cognitive**, and **psychiatric** symptoms.
- Average age at diagnosis is 40 years.
- Cognitive decline and behavioral changes can precede onset of motor signs by up to 15 years.
- **Executive function** is the primary cognitive domain affected.
- Psychiatric manifestations include depression, apathy, irritability, obsessions, impulsivity, paranoia, delusions, and hallucinations.
- Patients are often aware of deteriorating mentation.
- Increased rate of suicide (7%).
- Movement disorders include chorea (jerky, dance-like movements) and bradykinesia.

Diagnosis

- Extrapyramidal movement disorder in an individual with either a **family history** of HD or **genetic testing** that confirms an increased number of CAG trinucleotide repeats in the HTT gene.
- Mild or major NCD may be diagnosed prior to onset of motor signs if an individual is determined to be at risk based on family history or genetic testing.

Treatment

Symptom-directed therapy with **tetrabenazine** or **atypical (second-generation) antipsychotics**.

PARKINSON DISEASE (PD)

- An idiopathic, progressive neurodegenerative disease characterized by depletion of dopamine in the substantia nigra pars compacta (located in the basal ganglia).
- Up to 75% of patients with PD meet the criteria for major NCD, typically in advanced disease.

Clinical Manifestations

- Motor signs include muscular (lead-pipe or cogwheel) rigidity, resting tremor, bradykinesia, and postural instability.
- Cognitive manifestations consist of executive dysfunction and visuospatial impairments.
- Depression, anxiety, personality changes, and apathy are common.
- Psychotic symptoms, including visual hallucinations and paranoid delusions, may result from the disease itself or from adverse effects of the medications used to treat the motor symptoms.
- Prodromal symptoms and signs (e.g., micrographia, hyposmia, hypogeusia, constipation, personality changes, mood disorders, and REM-sleep behavior disorder) may occur up to two decades before motor abnormalities appear.

Diagnosis

- Diagnosis of PD requires the presence of **bradykinesia** and either **tremor** or **rigidity**.
- Associated with asymmetry of motor symptoms.
- Mild or major NCD is attributed to PD if **cognitive decline appears after the onset of motor symptoms** and no other underlying etiology is identified.
- Typically responds favorably to dopaminergic therapy.

Treatment

- Motor symptoms are most commonly treated with **carbidopa-levodopa** and/or **dopamine agonists**.
- High-frequency deep brain stimulation may lessen severe motor symptoms, but is associated with increased risk of depression.
- Cholinesterase inhibitors are used to target cognitive symptoms and may also ameliorate some of the neuropsychiatric symptoms (hallucinations).
- Psychotic symptoms may respond to a reduction in the dose of dopamine agonists.
- **Low-dose quetiapine** and **clozapine** are the preferred medications for treatment of psychosis. Avoid other antipsychotics since they can worsen the motor symptoms of PD.
- Pimavanserin is a serotonergic medication approved by the FDA to treat PD psychosis.

PRION DISEASE (TRANSMISSIBLE SPONGIFORM ENCEPHALOPATHIES)

- A form of subacute spongiform encephalopathy caused by *pro*teinaceous *in*fectious particles (prions).
- The most common type is **sporadic Creutzfeldt–Jakob disease (sCJD)**.
- Variant CJD (vCJD, aka bovine spongiform encephalopathy or mad cow disease) is a rare food-borne prion disease.
- Up to 15% are familial (autosomal dominant), involving prion protein (PRNP) gene mutations.
- Less than 1% of cases are iatrogenic.

Clinical Manifestations

- Insidious onset with **rapidly progressive** cognitive decline (over months to years).

KEY FACT

Symptoms of Parkinson disease can be exacerbated by antipsychotic medications.

KEY FACT

Rapidly progressive cognitive decline with **myoclonus** is suggestive of Creutzfeldt–Jakob disease.

- Presentation and progression vary by type.
- Typical clinical features of CJD.
  - **Myoclonus** (often triggered by startle response) is found in most individuals.
  - Visual (e.g., hallucinations, cortical blindness) or cerebellar disturbance (e.g., nystagmus, ataxia).
  - Pyramidal (e.g. positive Babinski sign, spasticity, hyperactive reflexes) or extrapyramidal dysfunction (e.g., bradykinesia, rigidity, dystonia).
  - Akinetic mutism in end-stage disease.

Evaluation

- Brain MRI: Hyperintensities in the caudate head, putamen, or at least two cortical regions on DWI or FLAIR.
- EEG: **Periodic sharp wave complexes**.
- CSF analysis: Positive RT QuIC assay and/or presence of 14-3-3 protein.

Diagnosis

- A diagnosis of probable sCJD requires either of the following scenarios:
  - A neuropsychiatric disorder with a **positive CSF RT-QuIC assay**.
  - **Rapid progression** of cognitive decline with two or more of the typical clinical features listed above AND typical findings on MRI, EEG, or CSF analysis.
- Definitive diagnosis requires analysis of brain tissue obtained via biopsy or autopsy.

Treatment

- No effective treatment yet available.
- Death usually occurs within 1 year of diagnosis.

NORMAL PRESSURE HYDROCEPHALUS (NPH)

- NPH is a potentially reversible cause of cognitive dysfunction.
- The etiology is either idiopathic or secondary to obstruction of CSF reabsorption sites due to infection (meningitis) or hemorrhage (subarachnoid or intraventricular).

Clinical Manifestations

- Classically presents with a clinical triad:
  - **Gait disturbance** ("Wobbly").
    - Most likely to be the first manifestation.
    - Slow with short steps.
    - Broad-based with outwardly rotated feet.
    - Feet appear to be stuck to the floor (magnetic gait).
    - Postural instability leads to recurrent falls.
  - **Urinary incontinence** ("Wet").
    - May begin as urinary urgency.
    - Gait disturbance may interfere with reaching the toilet before urinary incontinence.
    - In later stages, apathy may contribute.

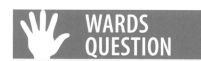

WARDS QUESTION

Q: What are the "three Ws" of NPH?
A: Wobbly (abnormal gait), **W**et (urinary urgency → incontinence), **W**acky (cognitive impairment).

- **Cognitive impairment** ("Wacky").
  - Insidious onset.
  - Executive dysfunction.
  - Psychomotor retardation.
  - Decreased attention.
  - Apathy.
- Enlargement of ventricles out of proportion to cortical atrophy on imaging.
  - **Localized elevation** of cerebrospinal fluid (CSF) pressure but **normal opening pressures** on lumbar puncture.
- Clinical improvement following CSF removal via lumbar puncture.

Treatment

- Placement of a shunt (usually ventriculoperitoneal) may improve symptoms.
- Cognitive impairment is least likely to improve.

NOTES

CHAPTER 9

GERIATRIC
PSYCHIATRY

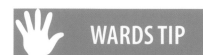

WARDS TIP

Work up an elderly patient for major depression when they present with memory loss or nonspecific physical complaints.

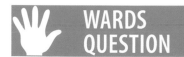

WARDS TIP

Patients with a major neurocognitive disorder are more likely to confabulate when they do not know an answer, whereas depressed patients may just say that they don't know. When pressed for an answer, depressed patients will often show the ability to answer correctly.

WARDS QUESTION

Q: What is the most common psychiatric disorder in the elderly?
A: Major depressive disorder.

The geriatric population of the United States is projected to more than double by the year 2050, boosted in a large part by the aging Baby Boomer generation. Nearly 20% of people over the age of 60 have a psychiatric disorder. The suicide rate of elderly (aged 85 and older) white men is five times the national average.

Common diagnoses in elderly patients include mood disorders, anxiety disorders, and neurocognitive disorders, though many psychiatric disorders in this population remain underreported and untreated.

Normal Aging

Factors associated with normal aging include:

- Decreased brain weight/enlarged ventricles and sulci.
- Decreased muscle mass/increased fat.
- Impaired vision and hearing.
- Minor forgetfulness (sometimes called age-associated memory impairment or benign senescent forgetfulness).

Major Depression

Major depression is a common disorder in the geriatric population, with depressive symptoms present in 5–15% of the elderly. Depression is associated with poor physical health:

- Post-myocardial infarction (MI) patients who develop depression have a four times increased rate of death.
- Stroke patients who develop depression have a greater than three times increased rate of death during the 10 years following their stroke.
- Patients with depression newly admitted to nursing homes have an increase in 1-year mortality rate.

Pseudodementia

Symptoms of major depression in the elderly often include problems with memory and cognitive functioning. Because this clinical picture may be mistaken for a major neurocognitive disorder (dementia), it is termed *pseudodementia.*

Pseudodementia is the presence of apparent cognitive deficits in patients with major depression. Patients may appear to be suffering from a neurocognitive disorder (dementia); however, their symptoms are secondary to their underlying depression, although it can be difficult to differentiate the two (see Table 9-1).

TABLE 9-1. Dementia versus Pseudodementia (Depression)	
Dementia	**Pseudodementia (Depression)**
Onset is insidious.	Onset is more acute.
Sundowning is common (↑ confusion at night).	Sundowning is uncommon.
Will guess at answers (confabulate).	Often answers "I don't know."
Patient is unaware of problems.	Patient is aware of problems.
Cognitive deficits do not improve with antidepressant treatment.	Cognitive deficits improve with antidepressants.

TREATMENT

- Supportive psychotherapy.

- Community resources: Senior centers, senior services, support groups, etc.

- Antidepressant medications (selective serotonin reuptake inhibitors [SSRIs] and other newer antidepressants have fewer side effects and are preferable to tricyclic antidepressants [TCAs] or monoamine oxidase [MAO] inhibitors).

- Elderly patients are sensitive to side effects of medications so it's important to start at a very low dose and titrate slowly up to the full dose of the antidepressant: "Start low and go slow!"

- If using TCAs in elderly patients, nortriptyline is favored because it has the fewest anticholinergic side effects.

- **At lower doses,** mirtazapine can increase appetite and be sedating; it is dosed at bedtime for depressed patients who particularly suffer from decreased appetite and sleep disturbances.

- Methylphenidate can be used at low doses as an adjunct to antidepressants for patients with severe depression and/or psychomotor retardation; however, it may cause insomnia if given in the afternoon or evening. Also, be aware of the risk of arrhythmia in patients with cardiac disease.

- Electroconvulsive therapy (ECT) may be used in place of antidepressants (ECT is safe and effective in the elderly).

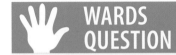

WARDS QUESTION

Q: What demographic has the highest rate of completed suicides?
A: White elderly males.

Mrs. Brennan is a 72-year-old female who considers herself to be in good health. She goes out to lunch with friends three times a week and looks forward to her Saturday bridge games at the local senior center. Unfortunately, her husband has suffered from years of ill health, including five myocardial infarctions and a serious stroke last year that left him barely able to walk. You are a geriatric psychiatrist who has been treating Mrs. Brennan's husband for depression that began after his last stroke. Mrs. Brennan always comes along to appointments so that she can stay informed about her husband's medical care.

You become concerned when your patient uncharacteristically misses an appointment and does not return your phone message. Finally, a month later, you are surprised to see Mrs. Brennan walk into your office alone. She enters the room slowly, and you notice that she has lost some weight since you last saw her.

She sits down but does not make eye contact. Finally, she begins to talk in a soft, monotone voice, explaining that her husband had another stroke last month and was moved to a hospice facility, where he passed away 2 weeks ago. She begins to cry, and you hand her some tissues. The two of you talk some more about her husband's death and how she is coping with it. She reports that her daughter visits her frequently and has invited her to spend the weekends with her.

Although Mrs. Brennan reports that she feels "down," she reports that she is making an effort to go on with her life because that is what her husband would have wanted. She says that she went out to lunch with her friends this week and adds that they are very supportive. Mrs. Brennan also reports that it is difficult for her to realize that her husband is no longer there and says that she has heard his voice calling her a couple of times this week. As she leaves your office, you tell her she is welcome to come back whenever she wants.

Is Mrs. Brennan having a normal grief reaction?

Yes, Mrs. Brennan is going through a normal grieving process, also known as bereavement. Although she displays some symptoms suggestive of major depression (psychomotor retardation, depressed mood), and reports the presence of auditory hallucinations (her husband's voice), these symptoms are commonly encountered in bereavement and are considered a normal reaction to her sudden loss.

Three months later, you receive a phone call from Mrs. Brennan's daughter, who expresses concern about her mother. She tells you that her mother has to be urged to shower, wear clean clothes, and eat regularly. Mrs. Brennan has stopped participating in her bridge group and has not been out with her friends in many weeks. The daughter also worries about Mrs. Brennan's increasing forgetfulness and memory problems. She asks if she can bring her in for an appointment with you. You agree and schedule Mrs. Brennan the next day.

Mrs. Brennan enters your office with her daughter by her side. She is dressed in a wrinkled pantsuit and is wearing scuffed shoes. Her hair is clean but lies limply against her head. She appears much thinner than the last time you saw her. Her eyes are downcast, and she appears sad. You try to engage her in conversation, but her answers to your questions are soft and short. When you do an assessment of her memory, you note that she answers basic questions with "I don't know" and scores poorly on the mini-mental state exam questions.

What is Mrs. Brennan's most likely diagnosis now?

Mrs. Brennan is most likely suffering from a major depressive episode. Her symptoms now fulfill criteria for major depressive disorder and have been present for over 2 weeks. Since her memory problems began after she began experiencing depressive symptoms, these are likely secondary to depression. When this occurs, it is often referred to as "pseudodementia." If this is the case, as her depression is treated her memory deficits will improve.

What are possible treatment options for Mrs. Brennan?

Supportive psychotherapy and a medication trial of an SSRI would be excellent first-line treatments. In addition, you suggest to Mrs. Brennan and her daughter to consider visiting her local senior center to learn what kinds of services from which she might benefit.

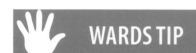

WARDS TIP

The elderly are very sensitive to side effects of medications, particularly anticholinergic effects of antidepressants.

Bereavement

In 1969, Elisabeth Kübler-Ross, MD, published a book called *On Death and Dying*, in which she proposed a model of bereavement, the Five Stages of Grief.

- **Denial:** *"This isn't happening to me. I don't feel sick."*
- **Anger:** *"It's my ex-husband's fault for smoking around me all those years!"*
- **Bargaining:** *"Maybe if I exercise and improve my diet, I'll get better."*
- **Depression:** *"There's no hope for a cure. I will die of this cancer."*
- **Acceptance:** *"I may have cancer, but I've always been a fighter—why stop now?"*

There is some controversy surrounding this model (e.g., people may not experience all of the stages or they may go through them in a different order) as grief is a very individualized experience; there is no "correct" way to mourn a loss. However, it is important to be able to distinguish normal grief reactions from unhealthy, pathological ones.

- **Normal grief** may involve many intense feelings, including guilt and sadness, sleep disturbances, appetite changes, and illusions/hallucinations (not always pathological in some cultures). These feelings generally abate within 6 months of the loss, and the patient's ability to function appropriately in their life is preserved.

- **Bereavement-associated depression** is a major depression that begins with a concrete death or loss in the patient's life. It is often difficult to distinguish between depression and grief, since many symptoms are similar.
  - Look for generalized feelings of hopelessness, helplessness, severe guilt and worthlessness, neurovegetative symptoms (e.g., insomnia, appetite/weight changes, low energy), and suicidal ideation, in addition to grief symptoms.
  - Treatment for depression is recommended in patients who have at least 2 weeks of persistent depressive symptoms.

Substance Use

- Forty percent of the 65 plus-year-old population drink alcohol, and up to 16% are heavy drinkers who may experience adverse health events from the amount of alcohol they use or from its interaction with medications and impact on chronic disease processes. It is important to screen elderly patients for substance use.
- Age-related effects of alcohol:
  - Elderly people have a lower amount of alcohol dehydrogenase in their livers which can lead to higher blood alcohol levels (BALs) with fewer drinks as compared to younger adults.
  - The amount of water in the body lessens with age, resulting in a higher percentage of alcohol in the blood of elderly compared to younger individuals after drinking the same amount of alcohol.
  - The central nervous system becomes more sensitive to alcohol with age.
- Chronic medical conditions worsened by alcohol:
  - Liver diseases (cirrhosis, hepatitis).
  - Gastrointestinal (GI) diseases (GI bleeding, gastric reflux, ulcer).
  - Cardiovascular diseases (hypertension, heart failure).
  - Metabolic/endocrine diseases (gout, diabetes).
  - Mental disorders (depression, anxiety).
- Alcohol and medication interactions (see Table 9-2).

TABLE 9-2. Alcohol and Medication Interactions	
Medication	**Result of Concurrent Alcohol Use**
H$_2$ blockers	Higher BALs
Benzodiazepines, tricyclics, narcotics, barbiturates, antihistamines	↑ sedation
Aspirin, NSAIDs	Prolonged bleeding time; irritation of gastric lining
Metronidazole, sulfonamides, long-acting hypoglycemics	Nausea and vomiting
Reserpine, nitroglycerin, hydralazine	↑ risk of hypotension
Acetaminophen, isoniazid, phenylbutazone	↑hepatotoxicity
Antihypertensives, antidiabetics, ulcer drugs, gout medications	Worsen underlying disease

Psychiatric Manifestations of Major Neurocognitive Disorders (Dementia)

Behavioral symptoms are quite common in patients with major neurocognitive disorders, and are often the source of many psychosocial problems surrounding their care. Agitation and aggression can be distressing and dangerous for caregivers, as well as unsafe for patients. Behavioral disinhibition is fairly common in major neurocognitive disorders and causes patients to act in ways that are quite unlike their typical behaviors (e.g., stripping off clothes in public, sexualized behavior, cursing).

■ Mood disorders:
  • Difficult to diagnose in a patient with confirmed major neurocognitive disorder.
  • Patients with major neurocognitive disorders may display many symptoms of depression (such as apathy) that are merely natural manifestations of their disease.
■ Aggression may be provoked by the following:
  • Patient's confusion in the setting of cognitive, memory, and language deficits.
  • Patient's inability to communicate discomfort or basic needs such as constipation, hunger, thirst, need to urinate, or pain.
  • Patient's hallucinations or delusions.
  • Patient with additional delirium
■ Psychosis:
  • Delusions are reported in up to 50% of Alzheimer patients.
  • Hallucinations (mostly auditory and/or visual) can be seen in at least 25% of patients with a major neurocognitive disorder.
  • If hallucinations do not bother the patient or interfere with caring for the patient, pharmacotherapy is unnecessary.

TREATMENT

Behavioral and environmental treatments for behavioral symptoms are much preferred in the elderly. Pharmacological methods are appropriate in the setting of potentially harmful behaviors, but care must be taken in dosing, duration of treatment, and interactions with other medications.

■ Nonpharmacological treatments:
  • Music, art, exercise, and pet therapy.
  • Strict daily schedules to minimize changes in routine.
  • Continual reorientation of patient.
  • Reducing stimuli (quiet living environments that are light during the day and dark at night).
  • Surrounding with familiar objects (family photos, a favorite quilt, etc.).
  • Ensuring patient has hearing aids, eyeglasses, and other basic needs.
■ Pharmacological treatments:
  • Antipsychotics:
    - Limited efficacy in treating agitation, and carry increased risk of mortality that must be discussed in a risk-benefit assessment with patient and caregivers.

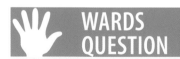

WARDS TIP

Visual hallucinations early in dementia suggest a diagnosis of neurocognitive disorder due to Lewy body disease. Antipsychotics should be avoided as these patients are sensitive to extrapyramidal symptoms (EPS).

WARDS QUESTION

Q: What is common condition in the geriatric population that can mimic depression?
A: Delirium.

- Try olanzapine (Zyprexa) or quetiapine (Seroquel) in patients with severe symptoms.
  - Can also use short-term haloperidol (Haldol) or risperidone (Risperdal).
  - Can be useful in psychiatric emergencies.
- Anxiolytics:
  - Anxiety symptoms may be due to unrecognized depression and respond well to an SSRI.
  - Reserve benzodiazepines for very short-term, acute episodes and remember to watch for disinhibition (paradoxical agitation) and worsening confusion.
  - Mood stabilizers: Few studies on their efficacy in the elderly.

Sleep Disturbance

The incidence of sleep disorders increases with aging. Elderly people often report difficulty sleeping, daytime drowsiness, and daytime napping.

- Outside of normal changes associated with aging (see Table 9-3), causes of sleep disturbances may include other medical conditions, drug/alcohol use, social stressors, and medications.
- Patients with movement disorders (Parkinson disease, progressive supranuclear palsy) have shallow sleep and may be more restless at night because of trouble turning in bed.
- Restless leg movements during sleep, likely due to a dopamine imbalance, are called periodic leg movements (PLMs).
- Nonpharmacological treatment approaches should be tried first (alcohol cessation, increased daily structure, elimination of daytime naps, encouraging daylight exposure, treatment of underlying medical conditions that may be exacerbating sleep problems).
- Sedative-hypnotic drugs are more likely to cause side effects when used by the elderly (memory impairment, ataxia, paradoxical excitement, and rebound insomnia) and increase risk of falls.
- If sedative-hypnotics must be prescribed, medications such as trazodone are safer than the more sedating benzodiazepines, but be careful of orthostasis.

Other Issues

RESTRAINTS

- In nonemergency situations, restraints should be used as a last resort and the patient should be reassessed at regular intervals.

TABLE 9-3. Normal Sleep Changes in Geriatric Patients	
Rapid eye movement (REM) sleep	↓ REM latency and ↓ total REM
Non-REM sleep	↑ amounts of stage 1 and 2 sleep, ↓ amounts of stage 3 and 4 sleep (deep sleep)
Sleep efficiency	↓ (frequent nocturnal awakenings)
Amount of total sleep	↓
Sleep cycle	Sleep cycle advances (earlier to bed, earlier to rise)

- Patient safety, health, and well-being should be the most important concern in the matter of restraint use.
- Evaluate ABCs in a restrained patient: airway, breathing, and circulation.

MEDICATIONS

- Many older people are on multiple medications ("polypharmacy").
- They suffer from more side effects because of decreased lean body mass and impaired liver and kidney function.
- When confronted with a new symptom in an elderly patient on multiple medications, always try to remove a medication before adding one.

ELDER ABUSE

- Types: Physical abuse, psychological abuse (threats, insults, etc.), neglect (withholding of care), exploitation (misuse of finances), and rarely sexual abuse.
- Approximately 10% of all people more than 65 years old; underreported by victims.
- Perpetrator is usually a caregiver (spouse or adult child) who lives with the victim.
- Physicians are mandated to report suspected elder abuse.

NURSING HOMES

- Provide care and rehabilitation for chronically ill and impaired patients as well as for those who are in need of short-term care before returning to their prior living arrangements.
- The majority of patients stay permanently, and fewer than half are discharged after only a short period of time.
- Careful medication review is imperative for nursing home patients who experience frequent hospitalizations and subsequent medication changes.
- Caregiver burnout is very common in families of these patients, and can negatively affect patient care.

Psychiatric Examination of a Child

SOURCES OF INFORMATION

Gather and integrate collateral information from multiple sources to obtain as accurate a clinical picture as possible: primary caregivers, teachers, pediatricians, and the child welfare system (if relevant).

METHODS OF GATHERING INFORMATION

Determine the child's **developmental stage** and tailor the interview appropriately.

- **Play therapy:** Utilizes the child's symbolic play, storytelling, or drawing as a forum for expression of emotions and experiences.
- **Classroom observation:** A window into the child's functioning in school.
- **Formal neuropsychological testing:** Quantitatively assesses a child's strengths and weaknesses by examination of their cognitive profile: intelligence quotient (IQ); language and visual-motor skills; memory, attention, and organizational abilities.
- **Kaufman Assessment Battery for Children (K-ABC):** Intelligence test comparing intellectual capacity with acquired knowledge of patients between 2 and 12 years old.
- **Wechsler Intelligence Scale for Children-Revised (WISC-R):** Assesses verbal, performance, and full-scale IQ of patients between 6 and 16 years old.

SAFETY ASSESSMENT

- Always screen for safety issues including self-injurious behavior, suicidal ideation, homicidal ideation, and command auditory hallucinations in a developmentally appropriate manner.
- In the United States, suicide rates have increased significantly and are currently the second leading cause of death in individuals 10–34 years old. In the United States, 2½ times as many suicides occurred as homicides. Collectively, deaths due to suicide and homicide have remained a major cause of premature death for victims between 10 and 24 years old.

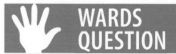

WARDS QUESTION

Q: Should you screen a new patient for suicidal ideation?
A: Yes. Asking a patient directly about suicidal thoughts may help save their life and does not cause suicidal tendencies.

Intellectual Disability

Intellectual disability (ID), or intellectual developmental disorder, is characterized by impaired cognitive and adaptive/social functioning. Severity level is currently based on adaptive functioning, indicating the degree of support required. A single IQ score does not adequately capture this and is no longer used solely to determine ID severity.

DIAGNOSIS AND *DSM-5* CRITERIA

- **Deficits in intellectual functioning** include learning, reasoning, judgment, planning, abstract thinking, and problem solving.
- **Deficits in adaptive functioning** include communication, social participation, and independent living.

- Deficits affect multiple domains including conceptual, practical, and social.
- Onset occurs during the developmental period.
- Intellectual deficits are confirmed by clinical assessment and standardized intelligence testing (scores at least two standard deviations below the population mean).
- Adaptive functioning deficits require ongoing support for activities of daily life.
- Severity levels: Mild, moderate, severe, and profound.

EPIDEMIOLOGY

- Overall: 1% of population.
- Severe ID: 6/1000.

ETIOLOGY

- Causes include genetic, prenatal, perinatal, and postnatal conditions (see Table 10-1).
- Fifty percent of ID cases have no identifiable cause.

Global Developmental Delay

- Failure to meet expected developmental milestones in several areas of intellectual functioning.
- Diagnosis reserved for patients less than 5 years old when severity level cannot be reliably assessed via standardized testing. Patients will need to be reevaluated when older to clarify the diagnosis.

Specific Learning Disorder (LD)

Characterized by delayed cognitive development in a particular academic domain.

WARDS TIP

Characteristic physical features of genetic syndromes:
- Down syndrome: Epicanthic folds, flat nasal bridge, and palmar crease.
- Fragile X syndrome: long, narrow face, joint hyperlaxity, and macroorchidism in postpubertal males.
- Prader–Willi syndrome: Obese, small stature, and almond-shaped eyes.

KEY FACT

Fragile X Syndrome Facts and Stats

- Most common inherited form of ID.
- Second most common cause of ID.
- Due to *FMR*-1 gene mutation.
- Males > females.

KEY FACT

Down Syndrome Facts and Stats

- 1/700 live births.
- Most common chromosomal disorder.
- Trisomy 21 = 3 copies of chromosome 21.

TABLE 10-1. Causes of Intellectual Disability	
Cause	**Examples**
Genetic	■ **Down syndrome:** Trisomy 21 (1/700 live births) ■ **Fragile X syndrome:** Involves mutation of X chromosome, 2nd most common cause of intellectual disability, males >females ■ *Other causes:* Phenylketonuria, familial mental retardation, Prader–Willi syndrome, Williams syndrome, Angelman syndrome, tuberous sclerosis
Prenatal	Infection and toxins (**TORCH**): ■ **T**oxoplasmosis ■ **O**ther (syphilis, AIDS, alcohol/illicit drugs) ■ **R**ubella (German measles) ■ **C**ytomegalovirus (CMV) ■ **H**erpes simplex
Perinatal	Anoxia, prematurity, birth trauma, meningitis, hyperbilirubinemia
Postnatal	Hypothyroidism, malnutrition, toxin exposure, trauma

DIAGNOSIS AND *DSM-5* CRITERIA

- Significantly impaired academic skills which are below expectation for chronological age and interfere with academics, occupation, or activities of daily living (ADLs).
- Begins during school but may become more impairing as demands increase.
- Affected areas: Reading (e.g., dyslexia), writing (e.g., dysgraphia), or arithmetic (e.g., dyscalculia).
- Not better accounted for by intellectual disabilities, visual/auditory deficits, language barriers, or subpar education.

EPIDEMIOLOGY

- Prevalence in school age children: 5–15%.
- Males > females affected.

ETIOLOGY

- Environmental factors: Increased risk with prematurity, very low birth weight, and prenatal nicotine exposure.
- Genetic factors: Increased risk in first-degree relatives of affected individuals.

COMORBIDITY

- Commonly co-occurs with other neurodevelopmental disorders, such as attention deficit/hyperactivity disorder (ADHD), communication disorders, developmental coordination disorder, and autism spectrum disorder (ASD).
- Comorbid with other mental disorders, including anxiety, depressive, and bipolar disorders.

TREATMENT

- Systematic, individualized education tailored to child's specific needs.
- Behavioral techniques may be used to improve learning skills.

Communication Disorders

Communication disorder includes impaired speech, language or social communication that are below expectation for chronological age. Symptoms begin in the early developmental period and lead to academic or adaptive issues.

- Language disorder—Difficulty acquiring and using language due to expressive and/or receptive impairment (e.g., reduced vocabulary, limited sentence structure, impairments in discourse). Increased risk in families of affected individuals.
- Speech sound disorder (phonological disorder)—Difficulty producing articulate, intelligible speech.
- Childhood-onset fluency disorder (stuttering)—Dysfluency and speech motor production issues. Increased risk of stuttering in first-degree relatives of affected individuals.

KEY FACT

Fetal Alcohol Exposure Facts
Fetal alcohol syndrome (FAS) = Leading *preventable* cause of birth defects and ID.
Three features of FAS:

1. Growth retardation
2. CNS involvement (structural, neurologic, functional)
3. Facial dysmorphology (smooth philtrum, short palpebral fissures, thin vermillion border)

Fetal alcohol spectrum disorders: Fetal alcohol exposure of any amount may cause a range of developmental disabilities, which are often underrecognized.

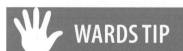

WARDS TIP

Always rule out sensory deficits before diagnosing a specific learning disorder.

■ Social (pragmatic) communication disorder—Challenges with the social use of verbal and nonverbal communication. If restricted/repetitive behaviors, activities, or interests are also present, consider diagnosis of ASD. Increased risk with family history of communication disorders, ASD, or specific LD.

TREATMENT

■ Speech and language therapy, family counseling.
■ Tailor educational supports to meet the individual's needs.

 A 10-year-old girl is referred for psychiatric evaluation because of academic and behavioral issues over the last year. The student has an above average IQ and seems to comprehend class material. Her teachers share concerns that she makes careless mistakes on homework and rushes through tests, leading to lower than predicted grades. She also blurts out answers without waiting for her turn. During the interview, she has difficulty staying focused and asks the examiner to repeat the question several times. Her mother complains that she does not clean her room or complete assigned chores.

What is the most likely diagnosis?
The patient has classic symptoms of attention deficit/hyperactivity disorder (ADHD) occurring in two different settings (home and school).

What treatment is indicated?

If the child does not have any contraindications, stimulant medications are usually the first-line treatment for ADHD.

Attention Deficit/Hyperactivity Disorder (ADHD)

ADHD is characterized by persistent **inattention**, **hyperactivity**, and **impulsivity** inconsistent with the patient's developmental stage. There are three subcategories of ADHD: predominantly inattentive type, predominantly hyperactive/impulsive type, and combined type.

DIAGNOSIS AND *DSM-5* CRITERIA

■ Two symptom domains: Inattentiveness and hyperactivity/impulsivity.
■ At least six inattentive symptoms:
  • Does not pay attention to details or makes careless mistakes.
  • Has difficulty sustaining attention.
  • Difficulty listening.
  • Struggles to follow instructions.
  • Is unorganized.
  • Avoids tasks requiring high cognitive demands.
  • Misplaces/loses objects frequently.
  • Is easily distracted.
  • Is forgetful.
And/or
■ At least six hyperactivity/impulsivity symptoms:
  • Fidgets with hands/feet or squirms in seat.
  • Has difficulty remaining still.

- Runs/climbs excessively in childhood (extreme restlessness in adults).
- Has difficulty engaging in activities quietly.
- Acts as if driven by a motor (an internal sensation in adults).
- Talks excessively.
- Blurts out answers before questions have been completed.
- Has difficulty waiting or taking turns.
- Interrupts or intrudes upon others.

■ Symptoms more than 6 months and present in **two** or more settings (e.g., home, school, work).

■ Symptoms interfere with or reduce quality of social, academic, and/or occupational functioning.

■ Onset **prior to age 12**, but can be diagnosed retrospectively in adulthood.

■ Not due to the physiological effects of a substance, *another medical or neurological condition (e.g., traumatic brain injury), or another mental disorder.*

EPIDEMIOLOGY

■ Prevalence: 10% of children and 4.5% of adults.

■ Males > females with 2:1 ratio.

■ Females present more often with inattentive symptoms.

ETIOLOGY

The etiology of ADHD is multifactorial and may include:

■ Genetic factors: Increased rate in first-degree relatives of affected individuals.

■ Environmental factors: Potentially in utero exposure to neurotoxin, low birth weight, or childhood abuse or neglect.

COURSE/PROGNOSIS

■ Stable through adolescence.

■ Many continue to have symptoms as adults (inattentive > hyperactive).

■ High incidence of comorbid oppositional defiant disorder, conduct disorder, and specific LD.

TREATMENT

Multimodal treatment plan: Medications are the most effective treatment for decreasing core symptoms, but should be used in conjunction with educational and behavioral interventions.

■ Pharmacological treatments:

- First-line: **Stimulants** (e.g., methylphenidate compounds, dextroamphetamine, mixed amphetamine salts).
- Second-line: Alpha-2 agonists (e.g., clonidine, **guanfacine**) can be used instead or as adjunctive therapy to stimulants. May be used in children who respond poorly to other medications, experience side effects, or have coexisting conditions such as tics.

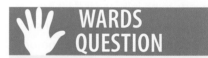

WARDS QUESTION

Q: What are first-line treatments in ADHD?
A: Stimulants.

- Second-line: Atomoxetine, a norepinephrine reuptake inhibitor. May be more appropriate when a history or family history of illicit substance use is present.
  - Nonpharmacological treatments:
    - Parental psychoeducation, parent management training.
    - Executive function coaching, behavior modification techniques and social skills training.
    - Educational accommodations such as classroom modifications.

Autism Spectrum Disorder (ASD)

ASD is characterized by impairments in **social communication/interaction** and **restrictive, repetitive behaviors/interests**. This disorder encompasses the spectrum of symptomatology formerly diagnosed as autism, Asperger's disorder, childhood disintegrative disorder, and pervasive developmental disorder.

DIAGNOSIS AND *DSM-5* CRITERIA

- **Problems with social interaction and communication:**
  - Impaired social/emotional reciprocity (e.g., inability to hold conversations).
  - Deficits in nonverbal communication skills (e.g., decreased eye contact).
  - Interpersonal/relational challenges (e.g., lack of interest in peers).
- **Restricted, repetitive patterns of behavior, interests, and activities:**
  - Intense, peculiar interests (e.g., preoccupation with unusual objects).
  - Inflexible adherence to rituals (e.g., rigid thought patterns).
  - Stereotyped, repetitive motor mannerisms (e.g., hand flapping).
  - Hyper/hyporeactivity to sensory input (e.g., hypersensitive to particular textures).
- Abnormalities in functioning begin in the early developmental period.
- Not better accounted for by ID or global developmental delay. When ID and ASD co-occur, social communication is below expectation based on developmental level.
- Causes significant social or occupational impairment.

EPIDEMIOLOGY

- Recent increase in prevalence to 1% of population. May be related to expansion of diagnostic classification and/or increased awareness/recognition.
- Ratio in males to females is 4:1.
- Symptoms typically recognized between 12 and 24 months old but varies based on severity.

ETIOLOGY

Etiology of ASD is multifactorial:

- Prenatal neurological insults (e.g., infections, drugs), advanced paternal age, and low birth weight.

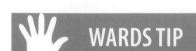

WARDS TIP

Consider ASD as the diagnosis if there is a rapid deterioration of social and/or language skills during the first 2 years of life.

Complete an appropriate work-up, such as auditory testing, prior to diagnosing ASD.

An extensive medical workup needs to be initiated if skills are lost after age 2, or more expansive losses occur (e.g., self-care, motor skills).

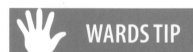

WARDS TIP

Assess for a potential cause of pain/discomfort if a nonverbal child with ASD presents with new onset aggression or self-injurious behavior.

- Fifteen percent of ASD cases are associated with a known genetic mutation.
- Fragile X syndrome = most common known single gene cause of ASD.
- Other genetic causes of ASD: Down syndrome, Rett syndrome, and tuberous sclerosis.
- High comorbidity with ID.
- Association with epilepsy.

PROGNOSIS AND TREATMENT

ASD is a chronic condition. The prognosis is variable, but the two most important predictors of adult outcome are level of intellectual functioning and language impairment. Only a minority of patients can live and work independently in adulthood. Treatment targets associated symptoms in order to improve basic social, communicative, and cognitive skills:

- Alpha-2 agonists (e.g., clonidine, **guanfacine**) and low-dose atypical antipsychotic medications (e.g., risperidone, aripiprazole) may help reduce disruptive behavior, aggression, and irritability.
- Early intervention.
- Remedial education.
- Behavioral therapy.
- Psychoeducation.

Tic Disorders

TOURETTE'S DISORDER

Tics are defined as sudden, rapid, repetitive, stereotyped movements or vocalizations. Although experienced as involuntary, patients can learn to temporarily suppress tics. Prior to the tic, patients may feel a premonitory urge (somatic sensation), with subsequent tension release after the tic. Anxiety, excitement, and fatigue can be aggravating factors for tics. Tics may present as simple or complex, depending on length of time, purpose, and orchestration.

Tourette's disorder is the **most severe** of the tic disorders. It is characterized by **multiple motor tics and at least one vocal tic lasting for at least 1 year**. Vocal tics may appear many years after the motor tics, and they may wax and wane in frequency. The most common **motor tics** involve the face and head, such as eye blinking and throat clearing.

Examples of **vocal tics**:

- *Coprolalia*—Utterance of obscene, taboo words as a bark or grunt.
- *Echolalia*—Repeating others' words.

Diagnosis and DSM-5 Criteria

- Multiple motor and at least one vocal tic present (not required to occur concurrently) for more than 1 year since onset of first tic.
- Onset prior to age 18 years.
- Not caused by a substance (e.g., cocaine) or another medical condition (e.g., Huntington disease).

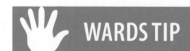

WARDS TIP

Tic disorders are one of the few psychiatric disorders in which diagnostic criteria do not require symptoms to cause significant distress.

Epidemiology

■ Transient tic behaviors: Common in children.

■ Tourette's disorder: 3 per 1000 school-age children.

■ Prevalence: Boys > girls.

Etiology

■ Genetic factors: > 55% concordance rate in monozygotic twins.

■ Prenatal/perinatal factors: Older paternal age, obstetrical complications, maternal smoking, and low birth weight.

■ Psychological factors: Symptom exacerbations with stressful life events.

Course/Prognosis

■ Onset typically occurs between 4 and 6 years, with the peak severity between ages 10 and 12.

■ Tics wax and wane and change in type.

■ Symptoms tend to decrease in adolescence and significantly diminish in adulthood.

■ High comorbidity with ADHD, OCD, and LD.

Treatment

■ Psychoeducation.

■ **Behavioral interventions**—Habit reversal therapy.

■ Medications—Utilize only if tics become severely impairing or also treating comorbidities. Due to the fluctuating course of the disorder, it can be difficult to determine medication efficacy.

  • Alpha-2 agonists: **guanfacine (usually first choice)**, clonidine.

  • In severe cases, can consider treatment with atypical (e.g., risperidone) or typical antipsychotics (e.g., pimozide).

Other tic disorders include:

■ **Persistent (chronic) motor or vocal tic disorder**: Single or multiple motor or vocal tics (but not both) that have never met criteria for Tourette's.

■ **Provisional tic disorder**: Single or multiple motor and/or vocal tics less than 1 year that have never met criteria for Tourette's.

WARDS TIP

A child may have **oppositional defiant disorder** if they no difficulty getting along with peers but will not comply with rules from parents or teachers.

Disruptive and Conduct Disorders

These disorders involve **problematic interactions** with or **inflicting harm** on others. While disruptive behaviors may appear within the scope of normal development, they become pathologic when the frequency, pervasiveness, and severity impair functioning of the individual or others.

OPPOSITIONAL DEFIANT DISORDER (ODD)

A maladaptive pattern of **irritability/anger, defiance, or vindictiveness**, which causes dysfunction or distress in the patient or those affected. These interpersonal difficulties involve at least one non-sibling (usually an authority figure).

Diagnosis and DSM-5 Criteria
Characterized by at least four symptoms present for more than or equal to 6 months (with at least one individual who is not a sibling):

KEY FACT

Unlike conduct disorder, ODD does *not* involve physical aggression or violating the basic rights of others.

- **Anger/Irritable mood**—Loses temper frequently; often angry and resentful.
- **Argumentative/Defiant behavior**—Breaks rules, blames others, argues with authority figures, and deliberately aggravates others.
- **Vindictiveness**—Is spiteful/vindictive at least two times in the past 6 months.
- Behaviors are associated with distress in the individual or others, or negatively impact functioning.
- Behaviors cannot be explained exclusively by the diagnosis of another mental disorder.

Epidemiology

- Prevalence: Approximately 3%.
- Onset usually during preschool years: Seen more often in boys before adolescence.
- Increased incidence of comorbid substance use and ADHD.
- Although ODD often precedes CD, most do not develop CD.

Treatment

- Behavior modification, conflict management training, and problem-solving skills.
- Parent management training (PMT) can help with setting limits and enforcing consistent rules.
- Medications are used to treat comorbid conditions, such as ADHD.

CONDUCT DISORDER (CD)

CD includes the most serious disruptive behaviors, which **violate the rights of other humans and animals**. These individuals inflict cruelty and harm through physical and sexual violence. They may **lack remorse** for committing crimes or **lack empathy** for their victims.

Diagnosis and DSM-5 Criteria

A pattern of **recurrently violating the basic rights of others or societal norms**. The individual has displayed at least three of the following behaviors exhibited over the last year and at least one occurring within the past 6 months:

- Aggression to people and animals: Bullies/threatens/intimidates others; initiation of physical aggression, including use of a weapon; robbery; rape; cruelty to animals.
- Destruction of property (e.g., fire setting).
- Deceitfulness or theft: Burglary; lying to obtain goods/favors.
- Serious violations of rules: Runs away from home, stays out late at night, and often truant from school before age 13 years old.

Epidemiology

- Lifetime prevalence: 9%.
- More common in males.
- High incidence of comorbid ADHD and ODD.
- Associated with antisocial personality disorder.

KEY FACT

Cruelty to animals may be indicative of **C**onduct disorder.

KEY FACT

Males: Higher risk of fighting, stealing, fire setting, and vandalism.
Females: Higher risk of lying, running away, sex-work, and substance use.

Treatment

- A multimodal treatment approach with behavior modification, family, and community involvement.
- PMT can help parents with limit setting and enforcing consistent rules.
- Medications can be used to target comorbid symptoms and aggression (e.g., SSRIs, guanfacine, propranolol, mood stabilizers, antipsychotics).

Elimination Disorders

Characterized by developmentally inappropriate elimination of urine or feces. Though typically involuntary, this may be intentional. The course may be *primary* (never established continence) or *secondary* (continence achieved for a period and then lost). Incontinence can cause significant distress or impair social or other areas of functioning.

DSM-5 DIAGNOSIS

Enuresis:

- Recurrent voiding of urine onto clothes or bed.
- Occurs two times per week for at least 3 consecutive months or results in clinical distress or marked impairment.
- At least 5 years old developmentally.
- Can occur during sleep (nocturnal), waking hours (diurnal), or both.
- Not due to a substance (e.g., diuretic) or *another medical condition* (e.g., urinary tract infection, neurogenic bladder, diabetes).

Encopresis:

- Recurrent defecation into inappropriate places (e.g., clothes, floor), which may be voluntary or involuntary.
- Occurs at least one time per month for at least 3 months.
- At least 4 years old developmentally.
- Not due to the physiological effects of a substance (e.g., laxatives) or another medical condition (e.g., hypothyroidism, anal fissure, spina bifida), except via a constipation-related mechanism.

EPIDEMIOLOGY

- Prevalence of enuresis decreases with age:
  - 5—10% of 5 year olds; 3—5% of 10 year olds; 1% of >15 year olds.
  - Nocturnal enuresis more common in boys; diurnal enuresis more common in girls.
- Prevalence of encopresis: 1% of 5-year-old children; boys >girls.

ETIOLOGY

- Genetic predisposition for nocturnal enuresis:
  - Approximately 4 times increased risk if history of maternal urinary incontinence.
  - Approximately 10 times increased risk if history of paternal urinary incontinence.
- Psychosocial stressors may contribute to secondary incontinence.

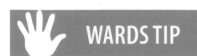

WARDS QUESTION

Q: What is the most common drug of abuse by adolescents?
A: Alcohol, followed by cannabis and vaping products.

WARDS TIP

The majority of enuresis cases spontaneously remit (5–10% per year) by adolescence.

- Encopresis: Often related to constipation/impaction with overflow incontinence.

TREATMENT

- **Psychoeducation** is key for children and their primary caregivers; provide information about high spontaneous remission rates.
- Treat if symptoms are distressing and impairing. Engage the patient as an active participant in the treatment plan. Encourage investment in a waterproof mattress.
- PMT for managing intentional elimination.
- **Enuresis treatment:**
  - Limit fluid intake and caffeine at night.
  - Behavioral program with monitoring and reward system, "bladder training" exercises, or **urine alarm** (upgrade from the **"bell and pad"** method).
  - Pharmacology can be used if the above methods are ineffective or for diurnal enuresis.
    - First line: Desmopressin (DDAVP), an antidiuretic hormone analogue.
    - Second line: Imipramine, a tricyclic antidepressant, can be used at low doses for refractory cases but has less tolerable side effects.
- Encopresis without constipation: Comprehensive behavioral program ("bowel retraining") for appropriate elimination.
- Encopresis due to constipation: Initial bowel cleaning followed by stool softeners, high-fiber diet, and toileting routine in conjunction with a behavioral program.

PANS/PANDAS

Pediatric acute-onset neuropsychiatric syndrome (**PANS** aka childhood acute neuropsychiatric symptoms or CANS) refers to a group of disorders characterized by the presence of **obsessive compulsive disorder** or **severely restricted food intake**. As suggested by the name, the onset is typically rapid, often described by parents as "appearing overnight." The presence of severe symptoms from two or more of the following categories are necessary to meet the diagnostic criteria:

- **Anxiety.**
- Emotional lability and/or depression.
- Irritability, aggression, and/or oppositional behaviors.
- Behavioral/developmental regression.
- Sudden deterioration in school performance.
- Motor or sensory abnormalities.
- Somatic symptoms and signs, including **sleep disturbances**, **enuresis**, or **urinary frequency**.

Pediatric autoimmune neuropsychiatric disorders associated with streptococcal infections (PANDAS) is a subtype of PANS. Diagnosis requires OCD and/or a tic disorder. The initial onset and/or periodic exacerbations are temporally associated with group A streptococcal infections. Motoric hyperactivity and/or adventitious movements are commonly present. While both PANS and

PANDAS have been topics of debate in regards to their etiologies, evaluation, and treatment, PANDAS is listed in the *DSM-5*, as an Obsessive Compulsive and Related Disorder due to Another Medical Condition.

Child Abuse

Child abuse encompasses physical abuse, sexual abuse, emotional abuse, and neglect. Toxic stress may result when children endure prolonged, severe trauma and adversity without the buffer of supportive caregivers. This can disrupt a child's development and lead to a spectrum of pathologic sequelae.

- About 1 million cases of child maltreatment in the United States.
- Up to 2500 deaths per year caused by abuse in the United States.

These numbers may be an underestimation as many cases go undetected and unreported.

PHYSICAL ABUSE

- Any act that results in non-accidental injury and may be the result of severe corporal punishment committed by an individual responsible for the child.
- Physical exam and x-rays may demonstrate multiple injuries not consistent with child's developmental age.
- Most common perpetrator is a first-degree male caregiver (e.g., parent, guardian, mother's partner).

SEXUAL ABUSE

- Any sexual act involving a child intended to provide sexual gratification to an individual responsible for the child.
- Sexual abuse is the most invasive form of abuse and results in detrimental lifetime effects on the victim.
- Data indicates approximately 25% of girls and 9% of boys are exposed to sexual abuse. Abuse is generally underreported, and males are less likely than females to report it.
- Children are most at risk of sexual abuse during preadolescence.

PSYCHOLOGICAL ABUSE

Non-accidental verbal or symbolic acts that result in psychological damage.

NEGLECT

- Failure to provide a child with adequate food, shelter, supervision, medical care, education, and/or affection.
- Victims of neglect may exhibit poor hygiene, malnutrition, stunted growth, developmental delays, and failure to thrive.
- Severe deprivation can result in death, particularly in infants.
- Neglect accounts for the majority of cases reported to child protection services.

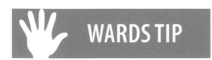

WARDS TIP

- Red flags for physical abuse: Delayed medical care for injury, inconsistent explanation of injury, multiple injuries in various stages of healing, head injuries, cigarette burns, spiral bone fractures, bruising patterns consistent with hand or belt.
- Red flags for sexual abuse: Sexually transmitted diseases, recurrent urinary tract infections, prepubertal vaginal bleeding, pregnancy, or trauma/bruising/inflammation of genitals/anus.

WARDS TIP

If a child reports sexual abuse, it should be taken seriously as it is rarely unfounded.

TREATMENT

Early intervention can potentially mitigate the negative sequelae and facilitate recovery.

SEQUELAE

- Increased risk of developing posttraumatic stress disorder, anxiety disorders, depressive disorders, dissociative disorders, self-destructive behaviors, and substance use disorders.
- Increased risk of continuing intergenerational abuse cycle with partners and children.

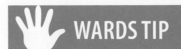

WARDS TIP

Doctors are *mandated reporters*, thus legally required to report all cases of suspected child abuse to the appropriate social service agencies.

NOTES

CHAPTER 11

DISSOCIATIVE DISORDERS

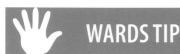

WARDS QUESTION

Q: When do dissociative responses typically occur?
A: During stressful and traumatic events.

KEY FACT

Dissociative amnesia refers to disruption in the continuity of an individual's memory. Patients with dissociative amnesia report gaps in the recollection of particular events, usually traumatic ones.

WARDS TIP

Patients suffering from dissociative amnesia can experience periods of flashbacks, nightmares, or behavioral reenactments of their trauma.

KEY FACT

Although dissociative fugue is now considered a subtype of dissociative amnesia disorder, it more commonly occurs in patients with dissociative identity disorder.

KEY FACT

Abreaction: The strong emotional reaction patients may experience while retrieving traumatic memories.

Dissociation can be understood as a **disruption in the integrated sense of self**. This may involve **lapses in autobiographical memory** (*amnesia*) and **feelings of detachment from one's self** (*depersonalization*) or from one's surroundings (*derealization*). These symptoms often develop in the context or aftermath of **significant trauma**, particularly **during childhood**. Dissociation may initially help buffer the impact of a trauma, but can also become pathological and maladaptive. While the dissociative disorders are closely related to the stressor- and trauma-related disorders, they are classified separately in the *DSM-5*.

Dissociative Amnesia

Individuals with dissociative amnesia are unable to remember important personal information or history, often **traumatic** in nature. **Procedural memory** (e.g., how to ride a bike) **is preserved**, distinguishing dissociative amnesia from other conditions resulting in memory loss (e.g., major neurocognitive disorders/dementias). The unrecalled autobiographical information has been stored in memory and is thus potentially retrievable. Dissociative amnesia rarely generalizes to encompass complete memory loss. More commonly, a single period of time (*localized amnesia*) or certain events (*selective amnesia*) are forgotten. Affected individuals often do not have insight regarding their deficits. There is a significant incidence of comorbid major depressive disorder or persistent depressive disorder (dysthymia) and an **increased risk for suicide**—particularly as amnesia resolves and the overwhelming memories return.

DIAGNOSIS AND *DSM-5* CRITERIA

- An inability to recall important autobiographical information, usually involving a traumatic or stressful event, that is inconsistent with ordinary forgetfulness.
- May present with *dissociative fugue*: **Sudden, unexpected travel away from home**, accompanied by amnesia for identity or other autobiographical information.
- Not due to the physiological effects of a substance, another medical or neurological condition (e.g., traumatic brain injury), or another mental disorder.
- Symptoms cause significant distress or impairment in daily functioning.

EPIDEMIOLOGY/ETIOLOGY

- Lifetime prevalence is 6–7%.
- Higher incidence in female patients.
- Amnesia often develops after trauma.

TREATMENT

- Important to establish the patient's safety.
- Psychotherapy (e.g., supportive, CBT, hypnosis) is the mainstay of treatment.
- Medications have not demonstrated efficacy in dissociative amnesia.

A 19-year-old male is found wandering several miles from home several days after a missing persons report was filed by his family. He cannot recall his full name or address, even when shown his ID card. His family reports that he recently returned from combat deployment.

Likely diagnosis?
Dissociative amnesia with dissociative fugue

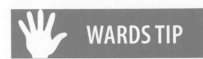

WARDS TIP

Fugue: Think of a *forgetful fugitive* who runs away and forms a new identity.

Depersonalization/Derealization Disorder

Characterized by repeated experiences of **detachment from one's self or surroundings**. Patients may feel as though they are observing themselves from a distance or have an **"out-of-body" experience** (*depersonalization*). They may experience the world around them as if **in a dream or movie** (*derealization*).

DIAGNOSIS AND *DSM-5* CRITERIA

- Persistent or recurrent experiences of one or both:
  - Depersonalization—Experiences of unreality or detachment from one's body, thoughts, feelings, or actions
  - Derealization—Experiences of unreality or detachment from one's surroundings.
- Reality testing remains intact during an episode, as opposed to during psychosis, when one cannot distinguish between what is real and what is not.
- The symptoms cause significant distress or social/occupational impairment.
- Not accounted for by a substance (e.g., drug of abuse, medication), another medical condition, or another mental disorder.

EPIDEMIOLOGY/ETIOLOGY

- Lifetime prevalence is 2%.
- Gender ratio 1:1.
- Mean age of onset is about 16 years.
- Increased incidence of comorbid anxiety disorders and major depression.
- Predisposing factors include severe stress and trauma.

COURSE AND PROGNOSIS

Often persistent but may wax and wane.

TREATMENT

- Psychodynamic, cognitive-behavioral, hypnotherapy, and supportive therapies may be helpful.
- There is a lack of evidence for use of medications to treat depersonalization/derealization disorder.

WARDS QUESTION

True or False? Transient experiences of depersonalization or derealization commonly occur in many otherwise healthy individuals.
True. Depersonalization and derealization can occur under stress, intoxication with substances, and even in benign circumstances (e.g., staring into a mirror for a prolonged period).

Dissociative Identity Disorder (Multiple Personality Disorder)

Dissociative identity disorder (DID) is characterized by the presence of **more than one distinct personality state** resulting from a fragmented sense of self. DID encompasses features of the other dissociative disorders, such as **amnesia**, **depersonalization**, and **derealization**. DID predominantly develops in **victims of significant and chronic childhood trauma**. Patients diagnosed with DID often cope with posttraumatic stress disorder (PTSD), depression, and suicidality.

DIAGNOSIS AND *DSM-5* CRITERIA

- **Disruption of identity** manifested **as two or more distinct personality states** dominating at different times. These symptoms may be observed by others or self-reported.
- **Extensive memory lapses** in autobiographical information, daily occurrences, and/or traumatic events.
- Not due to effects of a substance (drug or medication) or another medical condition.
- The condition causes significant distress or impairment in social/occupational functioning.

EPIDEMIOLOGY/ETIOLOGY

- Rare. No epidemiologic studies of the national prevalence, although a few community-based studies claim 1% prevalence.
- Increased prevalence in women.
- 90% of patients with DID have suffered from childhood physical abuse, sexual abuse, or neglect.
- Symptoms usually begin to manifest to some extent in childhood but may occur at any age.
- High incidence of comorbid PTSD, major depressive disorder, eating disorders, borderline personality disorder, and substance use disorders.
- More than 70% of patients attempt suicide, often with frequent attempts and self-mutilation.

COURSE AND PROGNOSIS

- Course is fluctuating but chronic.
- Worst prognosis of all dissociative disorders.

TREATMENT

- Psychotherapy is the standard treatment. Goals include maintenance of safety, stabilization, identity integration, and symptom reduction by working directly with traumatic memories.
- Pharmacotherapy: SSRIs to target comorbid depressive and/or PTSD symptoms (especially hyperarousal). Prazosin may ameliorate nightmares, and naltrexone may reduce self-injurious behaviors.

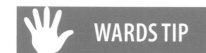

WARDS TIP

Symptoms of DID overlap with symptoms in borderline personality disorder or, to an extent, psychotic disorders.

A 21-year-old female is brought to the clinic by her boyfriend for evaluation of "memory issues." The patient recently visited her family for the holidays. The boyfriend states that "she had to deal with her abusive, alcoholic father. She seems like someone else ever since." The patient speaks in a childlike singsong voice and asks to be called by a name different than what is listed on her driver's license. She denies any concerns.

Most likely diagnosis?

Dissociative identity disorder (DID).

Other Specified Dissociative Disorder

Characterized by symptoms of dissociation that cause significant distress or impairment of functioning, but do not meet the full criteria for a specific dissociative disorder.

DSM-5 EXAMPLES

- Identity disturbance due to prolonged and intense coercive persuasion (e.g., brainwashing, cult rituals).
- Chronic and recurrent syndromes of mixed dissociative symptoms (without dissociative amnesia).
- Dissociative trance: An acute narrowing or loss of awareness of surroundings manifesting as unresponsiveness, potentially with minor stereotyped behaviors (not part of a cultural or religious practice).
- Acute dissociative reactions to stressful events (lasting hours/days → 1 month).

NOTES

CHAPTER 12

SOMATIC SYMPTOM AND
FACTITIOUS DISORDERS

Patients with somatic symptom disorders present with prominent physical symptoms; these are associated with significant distress or impairment in social, occupational, or other areas of functioning. While these patients may or may not have an associated medical condition, their focus is on their distressing somatic symptoms as well as their thoughts, feelings, and behaviors in response to these symptoms.

- Types of somatic symptom and related disorders include:
  - Somatic symptom disorder.
  - Conversion disorder (functional neurological symptom disorder).
  - Illness anxiety disorder.
  - Psychological factors affecting other medical conditions.
  - Factitious disorder.
  - Other specified somatic symptom and related disorder.
  - Unspecified somatic symptom and related disorder.

Up to 30% of primary care patients present with medically unexplained symptoms. In many cases, unspoken psychological needs manifest as physical symptoms. The symptoms may not make physiological "sense" but rather follow the patient's conception of how their body works.

 Ms. Thomas is a 31-year-old woman who was referred to a psychiatrist by her gynecologist after undergoing multiple exploratory surgeries for abdominal pain and gynecologic concerns with no definitive findings. The patient reports that she has had extensive medical problems dating back to adolescence. She reports periods of extreme abdominal pain, vomiting, diarrhea, and possible food intolerances. The obstetrician is her fourth provider because "my other doctors were not able to help me." Ms. Thomas reports fear that her current physician will also fail to relieve her distress. She was reluctant to see a psychiatrist and did so only after her obstetrician agreed to follow her after her psychiatric appointment.

Ms. Thomas states that her problems worsened in college, which was the first time she underwent surgery. She reports that due to her health problems and severe lack of energy, it took her 5½ years to graduate from college. She did better for a year or two after college but then had a return of symptoms. She reports recently feeling very lonely and isolated because she has not been able to find a boyfriend who can tolerate her frequent illnesses. She also reports that physical intimacy is difficult for her because she finds sex painful. Additionally, she is concerned that she might lose her job due to the number of days she has missed from work due to her abdominal pain, fatigue, and weakness.

What is the diagnosis?

Somatic symptom disorder. Ms. Thomas has a history of multiple somatic complaints lasting at least 6 months, along with a high level of anxiety about her symptoms and excessive time and energy devoted to her health concerns. She has had multiple medical procedures and significant impairment in her social and occupational functioning.

Somatic Symptom Disorder

Patients with somatic symptom disorder present with at least one (and often multiple) physical symptom. They frequently seek treatment from many doctors, often resulting in extensive lab work, diagnostic procedures, hospitalizations, and/or surgeries. Note that somatic symptom disorder and a related medical illness are not mutually exclusive.

DIAGNOSIS AND *DSM-5* CRITERIA

- One or more somatic symptoms (may be predominantly pain) that are distressing or result in significant disruption.
- At least one of the following:
  - Disproportionate and persistent thoughts about the seriousness of one's symptoms.
  - Persistently high level of anxiety about health or symptoms.
  - Excessive time and energy devoted to these symptoms.
- Persistent state of being symptomatic (typically >6 months; though the specific somatic symptoms may shift over time).

EPIDEMIOLOGY

- Incidence in females likely greater than males.
- Prevalence in general adult population: 5–7%.
- Risk factors include older age, fewer years of education, lower socioeconomic status, unemployment, and history of traumatic experiences in childhood.

TREATMENT AND PROGNOSIS

- The course tends to be chronic and debilitating. Symptoms may periodically improve and then worsen under stress.
- The patient should have regularly scheduled visits with a single primary care physician, who should minimize unnecessary medical workups and treatments.
- All treating physicians should recognize that the patient's suffering is genuine, whether or not there is an identifiable medical cause.
- Address psychological issues slowly. Patients will likely resist referral to a mental health professional.

Conversion Disorder (Functional Neurological Symptom Disorder)

Patients with conversion disorder have at least one neurological symptom (sensory or motor) which cannot be fully explained by a neurological condition. Examples include blindness, paralysis, and paresthesia. Patients may be surprisingly calm and unconcerned (*la belle indifference*) when describing their symptoms.

DIAGNOSIS AND *DSM-5* CRITERIA

- At least one symptom of altered voluntary motor or sensory function.
- Evidence of incompatibility between the symptom and recognized neurological or medical conditions.
- Not better explained by another medical or mental disorder.

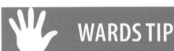

KEY FACT

Somatic symptom disorder patients typically express lots of concern over their condition and chronically perseverate over it. Conversion disorder patients often have an abrupt onset of their neurological symptoms (blindness, etc.) but appear unconcerned.

WARDS TIP

When treating a patient with a somatic symptom disorder, it is important for the psychiatrist to work closely with the patient's primary care physician.

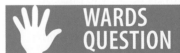

WARDS QUESTION

Q: Are patients with conversion disorder consciously faking their symptoms?
A: No. Patients with conversion disorder unconsciously produce symptoms, and cannot control when they occur. Symptoms may persist even after they become aware of their conversion disorder.

KEY FACT

Conversion-like presentations in elderly patients have a higher likelihood of representing an underlying neurological deficit.

- Causes significant distress or impairment in social or occupational functioning or warrants medical evaluation.
- **Common symptoms:** Paralysis, weakness, blindness, mutism, sensory complaints (paresthesias), psychogenic nonepileptic seizures (PNES), globus sensation (*globus hystericus* or sensation of lump in throat).

EPIDEMIOLOGY

- Two to three times more common in women than men.
- Onset at any age, but more often in adolescence or early adulthood.
- High incidence of comorbid neurological, depressive, or anxiety disorders.

TREATMENT AND PROGNOSIS

- The primary treatment is education about the illness. Cognitive-behavioral therapy (CBT), with or without physical therapy, can be used if education alone is not effective.
- While patients often spontaneously recover, the prognosis is poor: Symptoms may persist, recur, or worsen in 40–66% of patients.

Illness Anxiety Disorder

DIAGNOSIS AND *DSM-5* CRITERIA

- Preoccupation with having or acquiring a serious illness.
- Somatic symptoms are not present, or if present, are mild in intensity.
- High level of anxiety about health.
- Performs excessive health-related behaviors or exhibits maladaptive behaviors.
- Persists for at least **6 months** (the specific illness that is feared may change over time).
- Not better explained by another mental disorder (such as somatic symptom disorder).

EPIDEMIOLOGY

- Men are affected as often as women.
- Average age of onset 20–30 years.
- Approximately 67% have a coexisting major mental disorder.

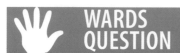

WARDS QUESTION

Q: In what setting are you most likely to diagnose a somatic symptom-related disorder?
A: Patients most commonly seek out care in medical settings—for example, primary care offices, medical specialty clinics, or emergency rooms. Patients are relatively unlikely to present to psychiatric settings, unless referred by a medical provider.

TREATMENT

- Regularly scheduled visits with one primary care physician.
- Psychotherapy (primarily CBT).
- Comorbid anxiety and depressive disorders should be treated with selective serotonin reuptake inhibitors (SSRIs) or other appropriate psychotropic medications.

PROGNOSIS

- Chronic but episodic—Symptoms may wax and wane periodically.
- Can result in significant disability.

- Up to 60% of patients improve significantly.
- Factors predicting better prognosis include fewer somatic symptoms, shorter duration of illness, and absence of childhood physical punishment.

Psychological Factors Affecting Other Medical Conditions

A patient with one or more psychological or behavioral factors (e.g., distress, coping styles, maladaptive health behaviors) adversely affecting a medical symptom or condition. Examples include anxiety worsening asthma, denial that acute chest pain needs treatment, and manipulating insulin doses in order to lose weight.

DIAGNOSIS AND *DSM-5* CRITERIA

- A medical symptom or condition (other than mental disorder) is present.
- Psychological or behavioral factors adversely affect the medical condition in at least one way, such as influencing the course or treatment, constituting an additional health risk factor, influencing the underlying pathophysiology, precipitating, or exacerbating symptoms or necessitating medical attention.
- Psychological or behavioral factors are not better explained by another mental disorder.

EPIDEMIOLOGY

- Prevalence and gender differences are unclear.
- Can occur across the lifespan.

TREATMENT AND PROGNOSIS

- Treatment includes education and frequent contact with a primary care physician.
- SSRIs and/or psychotherapy (especially CBT) should be used to treat underlying anxiety or depression.

Factitious Disorder

Patients with factitious disorder intentionally falsify medical or psychological signs or symptoms in order to assume the role of a sick patient. They often do this in a way that can cause legitimate danger (central line infections, insulin injections, etc.). The *absence of external rewards* is a prominent feature of this disorder.

DIAGNOSIS AND *DSM-5* CRITERIA

- Falsification of physical or psychological signs or symptoms, or induction of injury or disease, associated with identified deception.
- The deceptive behavior is evident even in the absence of obvious external rewards.
- Behavior is not better explained by another mental disorder, such as delusional disorder or another psychotic disorder.

KEY FACT

Münchhausen syndrome is another, older name for factitious disorder with predominantly physical complaints. Münchhausen syndrome by proxy is intentionally producing symptoms in someone else who is under one's care (usually one's child).

- Individual can present themself, or another individual (as in factitious disorder imposed on another).
- **Commonly feigned symptoms:**
  - *Psychiatric*—Hallucinations, depression.
  - *Medical*—Fever (by heating the thermometer), infection, hypoglycemia, abdominal pain, seizures, and hematuria.

EPIDEMIOLOGY

- May be at least 1% of hospitalized patients.
- More common in women.
- Higher incidence in hospital and health care workers (who have learned how to feign symptoms).
- Associated with personality disorders.
- Many patients have a history of illness and hospitalization, as well as childhood physical or sexual abuse.

TREATMENT AND PROGNOSIS

- Collect collateral information from medical providers and family. Collaborate with primary care physician and treatment team to avoid unnecessary procedures.
- Patients may require confrontation in a nonthreatening manner; however, patients who are confronted may leave against medical advice and seek hospitalization elsewhere.
- Repeated and long-term hospitalizations are common.

Malingering

A 37-year-old patient claims that he has frequent episodes of "seizures," starts on medications, and joins an epilepsy support group. It becomes known that he is doing this in order to collect social security disability money. *Diagnosis?* **Malingering**. In contrast, in **factitious disorder**, patients look for some kind of unconscious emotional gain by playing the "sick role," such as sympathy from the physician. The fundamental difference between malingering and factitious disorder is in the intention of the patient; in malingering, the motivation is external, whereas in factitious disorder, the motivation is internal.

Malingering involves the intentional reporting of physical or psychological symptoms in order to achieve secondary (external) gain. Common external motivations include avoiding incarceration, receiving room and board, obtaining narcotics, and receiving monetary compensation. Note that malingering is **not** considered a psychiatric condition.

PRESENTATION

- Patients usually present with multiple vague complaints that do not conform to a known medical condition.
- They often have a long medical history with many hospital stays.

- They are generally uncooperative and refuse to accept a good prognosis even after extensive medical evaluation.
- Symptoms quickly improve or resolve once the desired objective is obtained.

EPIDEMIOLOGY

- Not uncommon in hospitalized patients.
- Significantly more common in men than women.

MANAGEMENT

- Neuropsychological testing can help to identify feigned or exaggerated cognitive symptoms. Assessments routinely include embedded validity measures and tests more specifically designed to catch malingering or low effort, such as the TOMM (Test of Memory Malingering).
- Work with the patient to manage their underlying distress, if possible.
- Gentle confrontation may be necessary; however, patients who are confronted may leave the hospital Against Medical Advice (AMA) and seek treatment elsewhere.

KEY FACT

Malingering is the *conscious* feigning of symptoms for some secondary gain (e.g., monetary compensation or avoiding incarceration).

Review of Distinguishing Features

- **Somatic symptom disorders:** Patients *believe* they are ill and do not intentionally produce or feign symptoms.
- **Factitious disorder:** Patients intentionally produce symptoms of a psychological or physical illness because of a desire to assume the *sick role,* not for external rewards.
- **Malingering:** Patients intentionally produce or feign symptoms for *external rewards.*

NOTES

CHAPTER 13

IMPULSE CONTROL
DISORDERS

Impulse control disorders are characterized by problems in the self-regulation of emotions and behaviors. The behaviors violate the rights of others and/or conflict with societal norms. Impulse control disorders are not caused by another mental disorder, medical condition, or substance use.

Core qualities of the impulse control disorders are as follows:

- Repetitive or compulsive engagement in behavior despite adverse consequences.
- Little control over the negative behavior.
- Anxiety or craving experienced prior to engagement in impulsive behavior.
- Relief or satisfaction during or after completion of the behavior.

Mr. Baker is a 27-year-old married accountant who arrives at the outpatient psychiatry clinic complaining of difficulty in managing his anger. He has no prior psychiatric history, but reports that he has had difficulty controlling his temper since adolescence. He reports that he is easily angered by small occurrences, such as his wife's failing to make coffee or a coworker's forgetting a pen at work. He reacts quickly and in a volatile way, describing it as "going from 0 to 60 before I know it." Mr. Baker feels that he is unable to control his anger; on several occasions he has thrown objects and destroyed property in fits of rage, and has made threatening statements to his wife and coworkers in the past year. Because of these incidents, one coworker has recently threatened to pursue legal action.

Mr. Baker describes these episodes as brief, lasting only 10–15 minutes, and feels embarrassed shortly after the episode has transpired. He is concerned he may lose his job because of his behavior, and he worries about the fate of his relationships. He rarely drinks alcohol, and denies any history of illicit drug use.

What is his most likely diagnosis?

Based on Mr. Baker's history, his most likely diagnosis is intermittent explosive disorder. However, it is important to recognize that impulsivity is a common characteristic of other psychiatric diagnoses, and these must be ruled out prior to diagnosing a patient with this disorder.

What would be your recommended treatment?

Treatment for this disorder usually involves medications to treat impulsive aggression. These include selective serotonin reuptake inhibitors (SSRIs)—fluoxetine being the most studied—and mood stabilizers such as anticonvulsants and lithium. Individual psychotherapy is difficult and has limited efficacy given the nature of the disease and lack of individual control. However, cognitive-behavioral therapy (CBT) has been used in the treatment of anger management. Group therapy and/or family therapy may be useful to create behavior plans to help manage episodes.

What are associated laboratory findings?

In some impulsive individuals, cerebrospinal fluid testing shows low mean 5-hydroxyindoleacetic acid (5-HIAA) concentration. There may also be nonspecific electroencephalographic findings or abnormalities on neuropsychological testing.

Intermittent Explosive Disorder

DIAGNOSIS AND *DSM-5* CRITERIA

- Recurrent behavioral outbursts resulting in verbal and/or physical aggression against people or property.

Either:

- Frequent verbal/physical outbursts (that do not result in physical damage to people, animals, or property) twice weekly for 3 months.

Or:

- Rare (more than three times per year) outbursts resulting in physical damage to others, animals, or property.
- Outbursts and aggression are grossly out of proportion to the triggering event or stressor.
- Outbursts are not premeditated and not committed to obtain a desired reward.
- Aggressive outbursts cause either marked distress or impairment in occupational/interpersonal functioning, or are associated with financial/legal consequences.
- Aggression is not better explained by another mental disorder, medical condition, or due to the effects of a substance (drug or medication).

EPIDEMIOLOGY/ETIOLOGY

- More common in men than women.
- Onset usually in late childhood or adolescence.
- May be episodic, but course is generally chronic and persistent.
- Genetic, perinatal, environmental, and neurobiological factors may play a role in etiology. Patients may have a history of childhood physical or emotional abuse or head trauma.

TREATMENT

- Treatment involves use of SSRIs, anticonvulsants, or lithium.
- CBT has been shown to be effective and is often used in combination with medications.
- Group therapy and/or family therapy may be useful to create behavior plans to help manage episodes.

Kleptomania

DIAGNOSIS AND *DSM-5* CRITERIA

- Failure to resist uncontrollable urges to steal objects that are not needed for personal use or monetary value.
- Increasing internal tension immediately prior to the theft.
- Pleasure or relief is experienced while stealing; however, those with the disorder often report intense guilt and depression.

KEY FACT

Low levels of serotonin in the CSF have been shown to be associated with impulsiveness and aggression.

WARDS QUESTION

Q: What conditions should be considered in the differential diagnosis for an adult with possible intermittent explosive disorder? **A:** Substance intoxication or withdrawal, antisocial or borderline personality disorders, neurologic disorders (e.g., TBI, seizures), ADHD, bipolar disorder, and psychotic disorders.

- Stealing is not committed to express anger/vengeance and does not occur in response to a delusion or hallucination.
- Objects stolen are typically given or thrown away, returned, or hoarded.

EPIDEMIOLOGY/ETIOLOGY

- Three times more common in women than men, though rare in the general population.
- Occurs in 4–24% of shoplifters.
- Higher incidence of comorbid mood disorders, eating disorders (especially bulimia nervosa), anxiety disorders, substance use disorders, and personality disorders.
- Higher risk of OCD and substance use disorders in family members.
- Illness usually begins in adolescence and course is episodic.

TREATMENT

Treatment may include CBT (including systematic desensitization and aversive conditioning) and SSRIs. There is also some anecdotal evidence for the use of naltrexone, which blocks reward pathways mediated by endogenous opioids.

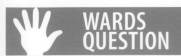

WARDS QUESTION

Q: What eating disorder is most commonly comorbid with kleptomania?
A: Bulimia nervosa. An estimated 65% of patients with kleptomania also suffer from bulimia nervosa.

Pyromania

DIAGNOSIS AND *DSM-5* CRITERIA

- At least two episodes of deliberate fire setting.
- Tension or arousal experienced before the act; pleasure, gratification, or relief experienced when setting fires or witnessing/participating in their aftermath.
- Fascination with, interest in, curiosity about, or attraction to fire and contexts.
- Purpose of fire setting is not for monetary gain, for expression of anger or vengeance, to conceal criminal activity, or as an expression of sociopolitical ideology. It is not in response to a hallucination, delusion, or impaired judgment (intoxication, neurocognitive disorder).
- Fire setting is not better explained by conduct disorder, a manic episode, or antisocial personality disorder.

KEY FACT

Pyromania is the impulse to start fires, typically with feelings of gratification or relief afterward.

EPIDEMIOLOGY/ETIOLOGY

- Rare disorder but much more common in men.
- Most begin to set fires in adolescence or early adulthood.
- High comorbidity with mood disorders, substance use disorders, gambling disorder, and conduct disorder.
- Episodes are episodic and wax and wane in frequency.

TREATMENT

Most don't go into treatment and symptoms will remain chronic. While there is no standard treatment, CBT, SSRIs, mood stabilizers, and antipsychotics have all been used.

CHAPTER 14

EATING DISORDERS

WARDS TIP

Suspect an eating disorder? Ask the patient what is their highest/lowest weight, their ideal body weight, if they count calories/fat/carbs/protein, how much they exercise, if they binge and purge, and if they have food rituals (e.g., drinking water between bites).

Definition

Eating disorders include anorexia nervosa, bulimia nervosa, and binge-eating disorder. Patients with anorexia or bulimia have a disturbed body image and use extreme measures to avoid gaining weight (vomiting, laxatives, diuretics, enemas, fasting, and excessive exercise). Patients with binge-eating disorder typically binge in response to negative emotions.

 Ms. Williams is a 17-year-old female without prior psychiatric history who is brought to the emergency room by ambulance after her parents called 911 when they found her having a seizure in their living room. She was admitted to the medical intensive care unit in status epilepticus and was quickly stabilized with intramuscular lorazepam and fosphenytoin loading. Her height is 5 feet 6 inches, she is of medium build, and her weight is 101 pounds (BMI 16.3 kg/m²). She has no significant medical history, and this is her first seizure. Laboratory workup shows an electrolyte imbalance as the most likely cause for her seizures. Although initially reluctant, she admits to self-induced vomiting several times this week. She reports that although she normally restricts her daily caloric intake to 500 calories, she regularly induces vomiting if her weight is above 100 pounds. Her last menstrual cycle was 1 year ago. Psychiatric consultation is requested in order to confirm her diagnosis.

As the psychiatrist on call, you evaluate Ms. Williams and find that she appears underweight and younger than her stated age. She is in mild distress, has a nasogastric tube in place, and exhibits poor eye contact. She reports feeling "sad" and admits to experiencing constant preoccupation about her physical appearance, stating "I'm fat. I hate my body." She also reports insomnia, low energy levels, and a history of self-harm behavior by cutting her forearms. She reports that she is careful in hiding her symptoms from her parents, whom she describes as strict disciplinarians. She also expresses concerns that she will disappoint them.

Ms. Williams's parents describe her as a perfectionist. They say that she is involved in multiple school activities, takes advanced placement classes, and has been recently concerned about being accepted to her college of choice. They report that she has maintained a 4.0 grade point average in high school, and they expect her to become a doctor. Her parents have noticed that she is underweight and rarely see her eat, but have attributed this to stress from her many academic pursuits. Ms. Williams's mother receives treatment for obsessive-compulsive disorder.

What is Ms. Williams's most likely diagnosis?

The most likely diagnosis is anorexia nervosa—binge-eating/purging type. As described above, she refuses to weigh more than 100 pounds, which is significantly below the minimal normal weight for her height. Despite being underweight, she expresses intense fear of gaining weight and has a disturbed self-image. In addition, she has engaged in binge-eating/purging behavior regularly. You should also explore for comorbid depression, anxiety, and a personality disorder. Remember that malnutrition in itself can lead to some of the symptoms experienced in depression, and that many patients show an improvement in their mood when nutrition is replenished.

What are some of the medical complications associated with this condition?

Patients with anorexia nervosa can present with bradycardia, orthostatic hypotension, arrhythmias, QTc prolongation, and ST-T wave changes on electrocardiogram, as well as anemia and leukopenia. They may also experience cognitive impairment, evidence of enlarged ventricles and/or decrease in gray and white matter on brain imaging, and peripheral neuropathy. Lanugo and muscle wasting sometimes become evident. Amenorrhea and loss of libido are commonly reported. In patients who regularly engage in self-induced vomiting, parotid enlargement, increased amylase levels, and electrolyte imbalances (e.g., hypokalemia) not uncommonly occur as a result, and may lead to seizures if severe.

Anorexia Nervosa

Patients with anorexia nervosa are preoccupied with their weight, their body image, and being thin. It is often associated with obsessive-compulsive personality traits. There are two main subtypes:

- **Restricting type:** Has not regularly engaged in binge-eating or purging behavior; weight loss is achieved through diet, fasting, and/or excessive exercise.
- **Binge-eating/purging type:** Eating binges followed by purges including self-induced vomiting, using laxatives, enemas, or diuretics. Some individuals purge after eating small amounts of food without binging.

DIAGNOSIS AND *DSM-5* CRITERIA

- Restriction of energy intake relative to requirements, leading to significant low body weight—defined as less than minimally normal or expected.
- Intense fear of gaining weight or becoming fat, or persistent behaviors that prevent weight gain.
- Disturbed body image, undue influence of weight or shape on self-evaluation, or denial of the seriousness of the current low body weight.

PHYSICAL FINDINGS AND MEDICAL COMPLICATIONS

- The medical complications of eating disorders are related to weight loss and purging (e.g., vomiting and laxative abuse).
- Physical manifestations: Amenorrhea, cold intolerance/hypothermia, hypotension (especially orthostasis), bradycardia, arrhythmia, acute coronary syndrome, cardiomyopathy, mitral valve prolapse, constipation, lanugo (fine, soft body hair typically found in newborns), alopecia, edema, dehydration, peripheral neuropathy, seizures, hypothyroidism, osteopenia, osteoporosis.
- Laboratory/Imaging abnormalities: Hyponatremia, hypochloremic hypokalemic alkalosis (if vomiting), arrhythmia (especially QTc prolongation), hypercholesterolemia, transaminitis, leukopenia, anemia (normocytic, normochromic), elevated blood urea nitrogen (BUN), increased growth hormone (GH), increased cortisol, reduced gonadotropins (luteinizing hormone [LH], follicle-stimulating hormone [FSH]), reduced sex steroid hormones (estrogen, testosterone), hypothyroidism, hypoglycemia, osteopenia.

EPIDEMIOLOGY

- Ten to one female to male ratio. Twelve-month prevalence among young females is 0.4%.

WARDS QUESTION

Q: What are the core differences between anorexia and bulimia?
A: Anorexia is marked by *low body weight* and restriction of caloric intake, while bulimia is marked by *normal* (or over) body weight.

KEY FACT

Classic example of anorexia nervosa: An extremely thin teenage girl with amenorrhea, whose mother says she eats very little, does aerobic exercise for 2 hours a day, and *ritualistically* performs 400 sit-ups every day (500 if she has "overeaten").

KEY FACT

Anorexia nervosa versus major depressive disorder: Appetite
Anorexia nervosa: Patients have a *good appetite* but starve themselves due to distorted body image. They are often quite preoccupied with food (e.g., preparing it for others) but do not eat it themselves.
Major depressive disorder: Patients usually have *poor appetite,* which leads to weight loss. These patients have no or decreased interest in food.

KEY FACT

Refeeding syndrome refers to dangerous electrolyte and fluid shifts that occur when severely malnourished patients are refed too quickly. Look for fluid retention and decreased levels of phosphorus, magnesium, and calcium. Complications include arrhythmias, respiratory failure, delirium, and seizures. Manage by replacing electrolytes and slowing the feedings.

WARDS TIP

When a patient with anorexia learns that weight gain is a common side effect, they may refuse medication.

- Bimodal age of onset (age 13–14: hormonal influences; age 17–18: environmental influences). More common in industrialized countries where food is abundant and a thin body ideal is held.
- Common in sports that involve thinness, revealing attire, subjective judging, and weight classes (e.g., running, ballet, wrestling, diving, cheerleading, figure skating).

ETIOLOGY

- Multifactorial.
- Genetics: Higher concordance in monozygotic than dizygotic twin studies.
- Social theories: Exaggeration of social values (achievement, control, and perfectionism), idealization of thin body and prepubescent appearance in Western cultures, increased prevalence of dieting at earlier ages.

DIFFERENTIAL DIAGNOSIS

- Medical conditions: Endocrine disorders (e.g., hypothalamic disease, diabetes mellitus, hyperthyroidism), gastrointestinal illnesses (e.g., malabsorption, inflammatory bowel disease), genetic disorders (e.g., Turner syndrome, Gaucher disease), cancer, AIDS.
- Psychiatric disorders: Major depression, bulimia, or other disorders (such as somatic symptom disorder or schizophrenia).

COURSE AND PROGNOSIS

- Chronic and relapsing illness. Variable course—may completely recover, have fluctuating symptoms with relapses, or progressively deteriorate. Most remit within 5 years.
- Mortality rate is cumulative and approximately 5% per decade due to starvation, **suicide**, or cardiac failure. Rates of suicide are approximately 12 per 100,000 per year.

TREATMENT

- Food is the best medicine.
- Patients may be treated as outpatients unless they are dangerously below ideal body weight (>20–25% below) or if there are serious medical or psychiatric complications, in which case they should be hospitalized for supervised refeeding.
- Treatment involves cognitive-behavioral therapy, family therapy (e.g., Maudsley approach—the gold standard for treatment of anorexia nervosa in teenagers), and supervised weight-gain programs.
- Selective serotonin reuptake inhibitors (SSRIs) have not been effective in the treatment of anorexia nervosa but may be used for comorbid anxiety or depression.
- Little evidence that second-generation antipsychotics can treat preoccupation with weight and food, or independently promote weight gain. Olanzapine has the most evidence in this regard.
- There is some consensus that a premeal anxiolytic (such as alprazolam) can help encourage eating by decreasing anticipatory anxiety.

Bulimia Nervosa

Bulimia nervosa involves binge eating combined with behaviors intended to counteract weight gain, such as vomiting; use of laxatives, enemas, or diuretics; fasting; or excessive exercise. Patients are embarrassed by their binge eating and are overly concerned with body weight. However, unlike patients with anorexia, they usually maintain a normal weight (and may be overweight).

DIAGNOSIS AND *DSM-5* CRITERIA

- Recurrent episodes of binge eating.
- Recurrent, inappropriate attempts to compensate for overeating and prevent weight gain (such as laxative abuse, vomiting, diuretics, fasting, or excessive exercise).
- The binge eating and compensatory behaviors occur at least once a week for 3 months.
- Perception of self-worth is excessively influenced by body weight and shape.
- Does not occur exclusively during an episode of anorexia nervosa.

PHYSICAL FINDINGS AND MEDICAL COMPLICATIONS

- Patients with anorexia and bulimia may have similar medical complications related to weight loss and vomiting.
- Physical manifestations: Salivary gland enlargement (sialadenosis), dental erosion/caries, esophageal tear or ruptures, callouses/abrasions on dorsum of hand ("Russell's sign" from self-induced vomiting), petechiae, peripheral edema, aspiration.
- Laboratory/Imaging abnormalities: Hypochloremic hypokalemic alkalosis, metabolic acidosis (laxative abuse), elevated bicarbonate (compensation), hypernatremia, increased BUN, increased amylase, altered thyroid hormone, esophagitis.

EPIDEMIOLOGY

- Twelve-month prevalence in young females is 1–1.5%.
- Significantly more common in women than men (10:1 ratio).
- Onset is in late adolescence or early adulthood.
- More common in developed countries.
- High incidence of comorbid mood disorders, anxiety disorders, impulse control disorders, substance use, prior physical/sexual abuse, as well as increased prevalence of borderline personality disorder.

ETIOLOGY

- Multifactorial, with similar factors as for anorexia (e.g., genetic and social theories).
- Childhood obesity and early pubertal maturation increase risk for bulimia nervosa.

COURSE AND PROGNOSIS

- Chronic and relapsing illness.
- Better prognosis than anorexia nervosa.

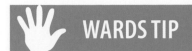

WARDS TIP

Unlike patients with anorexia nervosa, bulimic patients usually maintain a normal weight (or are overweight) and their symptoms are more ego-dystonic (distressing); they are therefore more likely to seek help.

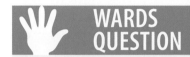

WARDS QUESTION

Q: What is binge eating?
A: Excessive food intake within a 2-hour period accompanied by a sense of lack of control.

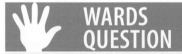

WARDS QUESTION

Q: What is a potentially lethal complication of both anorexia nervosa and bulimia nervosa?
A: Cardiac arrhythmias due to electrolyte disturbances such as hypokalemia.

KEY FACT

Compared to patients with bulimia nervosa, cortisol is often increased in patients with anorexia nervosa.

KEY FACT

Classic example of bulimia nervosa: A 20-year-old college student is referred by her dentist because of multiple dental caries. She is normal weight for her height but feels that "she needs to lose 15 pounds." She reluctantly admits to eating large quantities of food in a short period of time and then inducing vomiting.

WARDS QUESTION

Q: What is the only FDA-approved medication for the treatment of bulimia?
A: Fluoxetine.

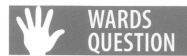

KEY FACT

In patients with bulimia, make sure to check that they aren't on medications that could further lower their seizure threshold, such as the antidepressant Wellbutrin (bupropion).

- Symptoms are usually exacerbated by stressful conditions.
- One-half recover fully with treatment; the other half have a chronic course with fluctuating symptoms.
- Crude mortality rate is 2% per decade.
- Elevated suicide risk compared to the general population.

TREATMENT

- Antidepressants plus therapy are more efficacious for treating bulimia nervosa than either treatment alone.
- SSRIs are first-line medication.
- Fluoxetine is the only Food and Drug Administration (FDA)-approved medication for bulimia (60–80 mg/day).
- Nutritional counseling and education.
- Therapy includes cognitive-behavioral therapy, interpersonal psychotherapy, group therapy, and family therapy. Cognitive behavioral therapy has demonstrated more efficacy than the other therapies.
- Avoid bupropion due to its potential side effect to lower seizure threshold.

Key Differences: Anorexia vs. Bulimia		
	Anorexia Nervosa	**Bulimia Nervosa**
Main concern	Concern about body weight with intense fear of gaining weight	Concern about body weight
Eating behavior	Avoids eating (restricting), ± purging	Binge eating with compensatory behavior (purging, exercise)
Weight	Underweight	Normal weight/Overweight
Medical complications	Nutritional deficiencies Hypotension	Nutritional deficiencies Russel's sign Dental/esophageal problems

Binge-Eating Disorder

Patients with binge-eating disorder suffer emotional distress over their binge eating, but they do not try to control their weight by purging or restricting calories, as do individuals with anorexia or bulimia. Unlike in anorexia and bulimia, patients with binge-eating disorder are not as fixated on their body shape and weight.

DIAGNOSIS AND *DSM-5* CRITERIA

- Recurrent episodes of binge eating (eating an excessive amount of food in a 2-hour period associated with a lack of control), with at least three of the following: eating very rapidly, eating until uncomfortably full, eating large amounts when not hungry, eating alone due to embarrassment, and feeling disgusted/depressed/guilty after eating.
- Severe distress over binge eating.
- Binge eating occurs at least once a week for 3 months.
- Binge eating is not associated with compensatory behaviors (such as vomiting and laxative use), and doesn't occur exclusively during the course of anorexia or bulimia.

PHYSICAL FINDINGS AND MEDICAL COMPLICATIONS

Patients are typically obese and suffer from medical problems related to obesity including metabolic syndrome, type 2 diabetes, and cardiovascular disease.

EPIDEMIOLOGY

- Twelve-month prevalence is 1.6% for females and 0.8% for males.
- Equal prevalence in females across ethnicities.
- Increased prevalence among individuals seeking weight-loss treatment compared to the general population.

ETIOLOGY

Runs in families, reflecting likely genetic influences.

COURSE AND PROGNOSIS

- Typically begins in adolescence or young adulthood.
- Appears to be relatively persistent, though remission rates are higher than for other eating disorders.
- Most obese individuals do not binge eat; those who do have more functional impairment, lower quality of life, and more subjective distress than weight-matched controls.
- Higher rates of psychiatric comorbidities than in obese individuals without binge-eating disorder.

TREATMENT

- Treatment involves individual (cognitive-behavioral or interpersonal) psychotherapy with a strict diet and exercise program coordinated by a registered dietician. Comorbid mood disorders or anxiety disorders should be treated as necessary.
- **SSRIs are first-line treatment due to their efficacy and tolerability.**
- Although not frequently used due to significant side effects and limited long-term efficacy, pharmacotherapy may be used adjunctively to directly promote weight loss:
  - Lisdexamfetamine (Vyvanse)—Stimulant that suppresses appetite and is FDA-approved for the treatment of binge-eating disorder.
  - Topiramate and zonisimide—Antiepileptics associated with weight loss.
  - Orlistat (Xenical)—Inhibits pancreatic lipase, thus decreasing amount of fat absorbed from the gastrointestinal tract.
  - Comorbid medical problems such as diabetes and metabolic syndrome should be monitored and treated appropriately.

NOTES

CHAPTER 15

SLEEP-WAKE
DISORDERS

Sleep disorders affect as many as 40% of the U.S. adult population. Current data demonstrate a high rate of comorbidity between sleep disorders and various psychiatric illnesses. Disturbances in sleep can potentiate and/or exacerbate psychological distress and other mental illnesses.

KEY FACT

As one ages there are the following changes that occur in the sleep pattern:

- Increase in time it takes to fall asleep, known as sleep latency
- Decline in total amount of REM sleep achieved
- Increase in sleep fragmentation with more frequent nighttime awakening

Normal Sleep-Wake Cycle

- Normal sleep-wake cycle is defined in terms of characteristic changes in several physiological parameters, including brain wave activity, eye movements, and motor activity.
- The two stages of normal sleep are rapid eye movement (REM) sleep and non-rapid eye movement (NREM) sleep.
- About every 90 minutes, NREM sleep alternates with REM sleep.
- NREM induces transition from the waking state to deep sleep.
- Progression through NREM sleep results in slower brain wave patterns and higher arousal thresholds.
- In REM sleep, brain wave patterns resemble the electroencephalogram (EEG) of an aroused person.
- Awakening from REM sleep is associated with vivid dream recall.

  See Figure 15-1.

Sleep Disorders

- Classified as either:
  - **Dyssomnias:** Insufficient, excessive, or altered timing of sleep.
  - **Parasomnias:** Unusual sleep-related behaviors.
- When taking a sleep history, ask about:
  - **A**ctivities prior to bedtime that may interfere with restful sleep.
  - **B**ed partner history.
  - **C**onsequence on waking function; quality of life.
  - **D**rug regimen, medications.
  - **E**xacerbating or relieving factors.
  - **F**requency and duration.
  - **G**enetic factors or family history.
  - **H**abits (alcohol consumption, use of caffeine, nicotine, illicit substances, and hypnotics).

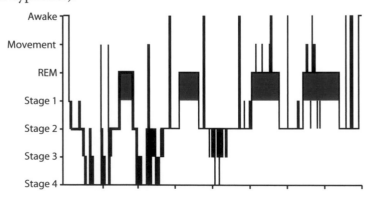

FIGURE 15-1. The sleep cycle. © 2008 LLS. Adapted, with permission of the publisher, Les Laboratoires Servier, from Figure 1 in Nutt D, Wilson S, Paterson L. Sleep disorders as core symptoms of depression. *Dialogues Clin Neurosci.* 2008;10(3):329–336.

Dyssomnias

Dyssomnias are disorders that make it difficult to fall or remain asleep (insomnias), or cause excessive daytime sleeping (hypersomnias).

INSOMNIA DISORDER

- Refers to a number of symptoms that interfere with duration and/or quality of sleep despite adequate opportunity for sleep. Symptoms may include:
  - Difficulty initiating sleep (*initial or sleep-onset insomnia*).
  - Difficulty maintaining sleep (*middle or sleep-maintenance insomnia*).
  - Early morning awakenings (*late or sleep-offset insomnia*).
  - Waking up feeling fatigued and unrefreshed (*nonrestorative sleep*).
- **Acute insomnia** (less than 3 months) is generally associated with stress or changes in sleep schedule and usually resolves spontaneously.
- **Chronic insomnia** lasts greater than or equal to 3 months to years and is associated with reduced quality of life and increased risk of psychiatric illness.
- **Diagnosis is often assisted by use of subjective sleep tracking measures such as the Consensus Sleep Diary.**

DSM-5 Criteria
- Difficulty initiating/maintaining sleep or early-morning awakening with inability to return to sleep.
- Occurs at least 3 days a week for at least 3 months.
- Causes clinically significant distress or impairment in functioning.
- Occurs despite adequate opportunity to sleep.
- Does not occur exclusively during the course of another sleep-wake disorder.
- Not due to the physiologic effects of a substance or medication.
- Coexisting mental and medical disorders do not adequately explain the insomnia.

Epidemiology
Prevalence: 6–10% (the most prevalent of all sleep-wake disorders).

Etiology
- Subclinical mood and/or anxiety disorders.
- Preoccupation with a perceived inability to sleep.
- Bedtime behavior not conducive to adequate sleep (**poor sleep hygiene**).
- Idiopathic.

Treatment
- Sleep hygiene measures.
- Cognitive-behavioral therapy (CBT) is the first-line treatment.
- Chronotherapy (bright light therapy) has evidence supporting its use in treating insomnia by entraining the circadian rhythm.
- Pharmacotherapy:
  - Benzodiazepines:
    - Reduce sleep latency and nocturnal awakening.
    - As effective as CBT during short periods of treatment (4–8 weeks); insufficient evidence to support long-term efficacy.

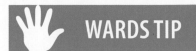

WARDS TIP

REM sleep is characterized by increase in blood pressure, heart rate, and respiratory rate.

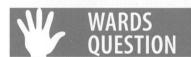

WARDS QUESTION

Q: What is the first-line therapy for chronic insomnia?
A: Cognitive-behavioral therapy; hypnotic medications are reserved for those who do not improve with CBT.

KEY FACT

Insomnia is the most common reason patients are put on long-term benzodiazepines.

- - Side effects include development of tolerance, addiction, daytime sleepiness, and rebound insomnia.
  - In the elderly, falls, confusion, and dizziness are of particular concern.
- Non-benzodiazepines:
  - Include melatonin, zolpidem (Ambien), eszopiclone (Lunesta), zaleplon (Sonata), and suvorexant (Belsomra).
  - Effective for short-term treatment.
  - Associated with low incidence of daytime sleepiness and orthostatic hypotension.
  - In the elderly, zolpidem causes increased risk of falls and may induce cognitive impairment.
  - Doses of zolpidem more than 10 mg can cause increase in cognitive impairment in women.
- Antidepressants:
  - Trazodone, amitriptyline, and doxepin (off-label use).
  - Mirtazapine (in low doses) is often used to promote sleep in patients with coexisting depressive disorders.
  - Side effects include sedation, dizziness, and psychomotor impairment.

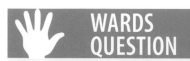

WARDS QUESTION

Q: What is the most common antidepressant prescribed for chronic insomnia?
A: Trazodone.

KEY FACT

Breathing-related disorders are the most common of the hypersomnias and include obstructive sleep apnea and central sleep apnea.

HYPERSOMNOLENCE DISORDER

- Refers to symptoms of excessive quantity of sleep, reduced quality of wakefulness, and sleep inertia/*sleep drunkenness* (i.e., impaired performance and reduced alertness after awakening).
- Complain of nonrestorative sleep, automatic behaviors (routine behavior performed with little to no recall), and difficulty awakening in the morning.

DSM-5 Criteria
- Excessive sleepiness despite at least 7 hours of sleep, with at least one of the following: recurrent periods of sleep within the same day; prolonged, nonrestorative sleep more than 9 hours; difficulty being fully awake after awakening.
- Occurs at least three times per week for at least 3 months.
- Causes clinically significant distress or impairment in functioning.
- Does not occur exclusively during the course of another sleep-wake disorder.
- Not due to the physiologic effects of a substance or medication.
- Coexisting mental and medical disorders do not adequately explain the hypersomnolence.

Epidemiology
- Prevalence: 5–10% of individuals presenting to sleep disorders clinics.
- Equal frequency in men and women.

Etiology
- Viral infections (e.g., HIV pneumonia, infectious mononucleosis, Guillain–Barré).
- Head trauma.
- Genetic—May have autosomal dominant mode of inheritance in some individuals.

Course

- Progressive onset, beginning between ages 15 and 25.
- Persistent course unless treated.

Treatment

- Life-long therapy with modafinil (first-line) or stimulants such as methylphenidate; amphetamine-like antidepressants such as atomoxetine are second-line therapy.
- Pitolisant (Wakix) and sodium oxybate (Xyrem) have shown benefit as well.
- Scheduled napping.

OBSTRUCTIVE SLEEP APNEA HYPOPNEA

Chronic breathing-related disorder characterized by repetitive collapse of the upper airway during sleep and evidence by polysomnography of multiple episodes of apnea or hypopnea per hour of sleep.

 A 40-year-old businessman states that over the past 2 years he has had trouble staying awake for more than 2 hours before eventually falling asleep. He then has a hard time sleeping through the night. As a result, his performance at work is suffering. *Diagnosis?* Many possible diagnoses, but you must always consider obstructive sleep apnea in addition to insomnia disorder, narcolepsy, etc.

Features

- Excessive daytime sleepiness.
- Apneic episodes characterized by cessation of breathing or hypopneic episodes of reduced airflow (more than 15 per hour).
- Sleep fragmentation.
- Snoring.
- Frequent awakenings due to gasping or choking.
- Nonrefreshing sleep or fatigue.
- Morning headaches.
- Hypertension.

Risk Factors

Obesity, increased neck circumference, airway narrowing.

Prevalence

- Most common in middle-aged men and women.
- Male to female ratio ranges from 2:1 to 4:1.
- Children: 1–2%; middle-aged adults: 2–15%; older adults: ⚁20%.

Treatment

- Positive airway pressure: Continuous (CPAP) and in some cases bilevel (BiPAP).
- Behavioral strategies such as weight loss and exercise.
- Surgery, including tonsillectomy and selective upper airway stimulation implants.

CENTRAL SLEEP APNEA

Evidenced by five or more central apneas per hour of sleep. It can be idiopathic, with Cheyne–Stokes breathing (pattern of periodic crescendo-decrescendo variation in tidal volume due to heart failure, stroke, or renal failure), or due to opioid use. It is associated with insomnia and daytime sleepiness.

Prevalence
- Idiopathic subtype rare.
- Cheyne–Stokes subtype increased in patients with decreased ejection fraction and acute stroke.
- Thirty percent of chronic opioid users have central sleep apnea.
- Higher frequency in men than women.

Course
- Tied to comorbid medical conditions, although may be transient.
- May be chronic in opioid users.

Treatment
- Treat the underlying condition.
- CPAP/BiPAP.
- Supplemental O_2.
- Medications (e.g., acetazolamide [Diamox], theophylline, sedative-hypnotics).

SLEEP-RELATED HYPOVENTILATION

Polysomnography demonstrates decreased respiration and elevated CO_2 levels. Individuals report frequent arousals, morning headaches, insomnia, and excessive daytime sleepiness. Frequently comorbid with medical or neurologic disorders, medication use, or substance use disorder. Over time it can result in pulmonary hypertension, cor pulmonale, cardiac arrhythmias, polycythemia, neurocognitive dysfunction, and eventually respiratory failure due to severe blood gas abnormalities.

Prevalence
Very uncommon.

Course
Slowly progressive.

Treatment
- Treat the underlying condition.
- CPAP/BiPAP.
- Medications to stimulate/promote breathing (e.g., bronchodilators, theophylline).

Mr. Richards is a 22-year-old college student with a history of persistent depressive disorder (dysthymic disorder) who arrives at the outpatient psychiatry clinic complaining of daytime sleepiness. He reports that during the past 2 years, he has fallen asleep while in social situations and during his college classes. He often takes naps during class, in movie theaters, and sometimes in the middle of conversations with his girlfriend. His naps typically last for 5–10 minutes and he awakens feeling better. However, within the next 2–3 hours he feels sleepy again. His colleagues joke about his tendency to sleep everywhere, and he feels embarrassed by this.

Mr. Richards also complains of "weird" experiences while sleeping. He reports that he sometimes sees bright colors and hears loud sounds that feel real to him. He says that when this occurs it is difficult to distinguish if he is dreaming or is awake. He feels frightened by these experiences because he is unable to move when they happen. However, after a few minutes he reports that these feelings resolve, and he is able to move and is fully awake.

In performing a thorough history, you learn that he has had episodes during which he has experienced weakness and has dropped objects from his hands while laughing or becoming angry. Last week, his legs buckled and he fell to the ground after his friends startled him at a surprise birthday party. He denies ever losing consciousness during these episodes, and there have been no reports of witnessed convulsions.

What is this patient's diagnosis?

This patient's symptoms are consistent with a diagnosis of narcolepsy. The classic narcolepsy tetrad (all four present in less than 25% of patients) consists of excessive daytime sleepiness or "sleep attacks," REM-related sleep phenomena including inability to move during the transition from sleep to wakefulness, hypnagogic or hypnopompic hallucinations, and a sudden loss of muscle tone evoked by strong emotion without loss of consciousness (cataplexy). Cataplexy may be mild, affecting only the voice, face, or arms, or generalized, causing patients to fall to the ground, and it occurs in 70% of those diagnosed with narcolepsy.

What are Mr. Richards's treatment options?

In the treatment of narcolepsy, it is important for patients to schedule daytime naps and to maintain a regular sleep schedule at night. They should get at least 8 hours of sleep and keep consistent times for sleeping and awakening. Pharmacological treatments may include the use of stimulants (methylphenidate) and antidepressants. The stimulant modafinil and sodium oxybate (nonstimulant) are also effective in the treatment of narcolepsy. Sodium oxybate (Xyrem) is particularly effective in the treatment of cataplexy.

NARCOLEPSY

Narcolepsy is characterized by excessive daytime sleepiness and falling asleep at inappropriate times.

DSM-5 Criteria

- Recurrent episodes of need to sleep, lapsing into sleep, or napping during the day, occurring at least three times per week for at least 3 months associated with at least one of the following:
  - Cataplexy (brief episodes of sudden bilateral loss of muscle tone, most often associated with intense emotion).
  - Hypocretin deficiency in the CSF.
  - Reduced REM sleep latency on polysomnography.
- Hallucinations and/or sleep paralysis at the beginning or end of sleep episodes are common (but not necessary for diagnosis in the DSM-5).

 KEY FACT

Hypnagogic hallucination: When going to sleep.
Hyponopompic hallucination: When transitioning from sleep.

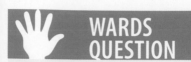

Q: What study is useful in diagnosing narcolepsy?
A: Polysomnography.

KEY FACT

Don't confuse narcoleptic cataplexy with catatonic catalepsy (unprovoked muscular rigidity).

Epidemiology/Prevalence
- Narcolepsy with cataplexy occurs in 0.02–0.04% worldwide.
- Slightly more common in males than females.

Pathophysiology
- Linked to a loss of hypothalamic neurons that produce hypocretin which has excitatory effects promoting wakefulness.
- May have autoimmune component.
- Secondary causes include lesions to the posterior hypothalamus and midbrain.

Treatment
- Sleep hygiene.
- Scheduled daytime naps.
- Avoidance of shift work.
- For excessive daytime sleepiness:
  - Modafinil is first-line pharmacologic treatment.
  - Amphetamines (D-amphetamine, methamphetamine).
  - Other non-amphetamines such as methylphenidate, sodium oxybate, and pitolisant (a novel histamine H3 receptor inverse agonist that is effective for both daytime sleepiness and cataplexy).
- For cataplexy:
  - Sodium oxybate (drug of choice).
  - Tricyclic antidepressants (TCAs): Imipramine, desipramine, and clomipramine.
  - **REM suppression drugs** such as selective serotonin reuptake inhibitor (SSRI)/serotonin-norepinephrine reuptake inhibitor (SNRI): Fluoxetine, duloxetine, atomoxetine, venlafaxine.
- **Sedative hypnotics are given in some cases to correct disturbed nighttime sleep.**

CIRCADIAN RHYTHM SLEEP-WAKE DISORDERS

Circadian rhythm sleep-wake disorders are recurrent patterns of sleep disruption due to an alteration of the circadian system or misalignment between the endogenous circadian rhythm and sleep-wake schedule required by an individual's environment or schedule. Subtypes include delayed sleep phase, advanced sleep phase, irregular sleep-wake, non-24-hour sleep-wake, and shift work (see Table 15-1).

KEY FACT

The suprachiasmatic nucleus (SCN) in the hypothalamus coordinates 24-hour or circadian rhythmicity.

Symptoms
- Excessive daytime sleepiness.
- Insomnia.
- Sleep inertia.
- Headaches.
- Difficulty concentrating.
- Increased reaction times and frequent performance errors.
- Irritability.
- Waking up at inappropriate times.

TABLE 15-1. Circadian Rhythm Sleep-Wake Disorders

Disorders	Definitions	Risk Factors	Treatments
Delayed sleep phase disorder (DSPD)	Chronic or recurrent delay in sleep onset and awakening times with preserved quality and duration of sleep	■ Puberty (secondary to temporal changes in melatonin secretion) ■ Caffeine and nicotine use ■ Irregular sleep schedules	■ Timed bright light phototherapy during early morning ■ Administration of melatonin in the evening ■ Chronotherapy (delaying bedtime by a few hours each night)
Advanced sleep phase disorder	Normal duration and quality of sleep with sleep onset and awakening times earlier than desired	Older age	■ Timed bright light phototherapy prior to bedtime ■ Early morning melatonin not recommended (may cause daytime sedation)
Shift-work disorder (SWD)	Sleep deprivation and misalignment of the circadian rhythm secondary to nontraditional work hours	■ Night shift work ■ Rotating shifts ■ Shifts >16 hours ■ *Medical and psychiatry residents*	■ Avoid risk factors ■ Bright light phototherapy to facilitate rapid adaptation to night shift ■ Modafinil may be helpful for patients with severe SWD
Jet lag disorder	Sleep disturbances (insomnia, hypersomnia) associated with travel across multiple time zones	Recent sleep deprivation	■ Disorder is usually self-limiting ■ Sleep disturbances generally resolve 2–3 days after travel

Parasomnias

- Abnormal behaviors, experiences, or physiological events that occur during sleep or sleep-wake transitions.
- Symptoms may include abnormal movements, emotions, dreams, and autonomic activity.
- Isolated episodes common in childhood and adolescence.
- Include non-REM sleep arousal disorders, nightmare disorder, REM sleep behavior disorder, restless leg syndrome.

See Table 15-2.

NON-REM SLEEP AROUSAL DISORDERS

Repeated episodes of incomplete arousals that are brief and usually occur during the first one-third of the sleep episode. Include sleepwalking and sleep terrors.

SLEEPWALKING

Features
- Repeated episodes of simple to complex behaviors that occur during slow-wave (NREM) sleep.
- Behaviors may include sitting up in bed, walking around, eating, and in some cases "escaping" outdoors.
- Eyes are usually open with a blank stare and "glassy look."
- Difficulty arousing the sleepwalker during an episode.
- Dreams are not remembered and there is amnesia for the episode.
- Episodes usually end with patients returning to bed or awakening (briefly) confused and disoriented.
- Rare cases associated with violent behavior.

TABLE 15-2. Comparison of REM and NREM Sleep Disorders		
	NREM Disorders	**REM Disorders**
Examples	■ Sleepwalking ■ Sleep terrors	■ REM sleep behavior disorder ■ Nightmares
Timing	■ Slow wave sleep ■ First one-third of sleep	■ REM sleep ■ Last third of sleep
Behaviors	■ Simple to complex (e.g., sitting, walking, eating)	■ Complex behaviors with gross motor movements, vocalizations (e.g., yelling, limb jerking, punching, kicking)
Recall and orientation upon awakening	■ Disoriented ■ Confused ■ Amnesia for the episode	■ Oriented ■ Vivid recall
Risk factors	■ Sleep deprivation ■ Stress ■ OSA ■ Medications ■ Seizures ■ Fever	■ REM sleep behavior disorder (RSBD): 　■ Older age 　■ Medications 　■ Narcolepsy 　■ Neurogenerative disorder ■ Nightmares: 　■ Adolescence and early adulthood 　■ PTSD

Epidemiology
- 1–7% of adults have sleepwalking episodes (not disorder).
- 10–30% of children have at least one episode and 2–3% sleepwalk often.

Risk Factors
- Sleep deprivation.
- Irregular sleep schedules.
- Stress.
- Fatigue.
- Obstructive sleep apnea.
- Nocturnal seizures.
- Fever.
- Medications, including sedatives/hypnotics, lithium, and anticholinergics.
- Family history.

Etiology
- Unknown.
- Family history in 80% of cases.
- Usually not associated with any significant underlying psychiatric or psychological problems.

Treatment
- Most cases do not need to be treated as they are self-limiting.
- Patients may benefit from education, reassurance, addressing precipitating factors, ensuring a safe environment, and proper sleep hygiene.
- Refractory cases may respond to low-dose benzodiazepine (e.g., clonazepam).

SLEEP TERRORS

Features

- Recurrent episodes of sudden terror arousals, usually beginning with screaming or crying, that occur during slow-wave sleep.
- Signs of autonomic arousal, including tachycardia, tachypnea, diaphoresis, and mydriasis.
- Difficulty arousing during an episode.
- After episode, patients usually return to sleep without awakening.
- Dreams are not remembered and there is amnesia for the episode.
- In rare cases, awakening elicits aggressive behavior.

Epidemiology

- Approximately 2% of adults and 20% of young children have sleep terrors (not disorder).
- Tenfold increase in first-degree biological relatives of affected patients.
- High comorbidity with sleepwalking.

Risk Factors

- Same as for sleepwalking.
- Other sleep disorder such as sleep apnea.

Treatment

- Reassurance that the condition is benign and self-limited.
- Same as for sleepwalking.

NIGHTMARE DISORDER

Features

- Recurrent frightening dreams that occur during the second half of the sleep episode (i.e., during REM sleep).
- Terminate in awakening with vivid recall.
- No confusion or disorientation upon awakening.
- Causes clinically significant distress or impairment in functioning.

Epidemiology

- Frequent nightmares in 1–2% of adults, higher prevalence in women.
- Peak prevalence in late adolescence or early adulthood.
- Nightmares are seen in at least 50–70% of posttraumatic stress disorder (PTSD) cases.

Treatment

- Not always needed. Reassurance may help in many cases.
- **Desensitization/Imagery rehearsal therapy** (IRT) involves the use of mental imagery to modify the outcome of a recurrent nightmare, writing down the improved outcome, and then mentally rehearsing it in a relaxed state.
- **Medications are rarely indicated**. Prazosin and antidepressants are often used to treat nightmares related to PTSD.

KEY FACT

Imagery rehearsal therapy (IRT) has been successful in treating recurrent nightmares in patients with PTSD.

REM SLEEP BEHAVIOR DISORDER

Features

- Repeated arousals during sleep associated with vocalization or complex motor behavior (dream-enacting behaviors) occurring during REM, more often in the second half of the sleep episode.
- Characterized by lack of normal muscle atonia during REM sleep.
- No confusion or disorientation upon awakening.
- Dream-enacting behaviors include:
  - Sleep talking.
  - Yelling.
  - Limb jerking.
  - Walking and/or running.
  - Punching and/or other violent behaviors.
- Presenting complaint is often violent behaviors during sleep resulting in injury to the patient and/or to the bed partner.

Epidemiology

- Prevalence in general population is approximately 0.5%, likely higher in people with psychiatric disorders.
- Occurs mostly in males.

Risk Factors

- Older age, generally more than 50 years.
- Psychiatric medications such as TCAs, SSRIs, SNRIs, and β-blockers.
- Narcolepsy.
- Highly associated with underlying neurodegenerative disorders, especially Parkinson, multiple system atrophy, and neurocognitive disorder with Lewy bodies.

Treatment

- Discontinuation of likely causative medications if possible.
- Clonazepam is efficacious in most patients.
- Melatonin may also be helpful.
- Ensure environmental safety such as removing potentially dangerous objects from the bedroom and sleeping on the ground until behaviors can be managed effectively.

WARDS QUESTION

Q: Which neurocognitive disorder is commonly associated with REM sleep behavior disorder?

A: Neurocognitive disorder with Lewy bodies.

RESTLESS LEGS SYNDROME

Features

The urge to move legs accompanied by unpleasant sensation in the legs, characterized by relief with movement, aggravation with inactivity, and only occurring or worsening in the evening.

Epidemiology

- Prevalence is 2–7% in the general population.
- Females 1.5–2 times more likely than males.

Risk Factors

- Increases with age.
- Strong familial component.
- Iron deficiency.
- Antidepressants, antipsychotics, dopamine-blocking antiemetics, and antihistamines can contribute to or worsen symptoms.
- Multiple medical comorbidities, including cardiovascular disease, diabetes mellitus, chronic kidney disease, and Parkinson disease.

Treatment

- Behavioral strategies including regular exercise, reduced caffeine intake, and avoiding aggravating factors have been shown to be beneficial.
- Responds well to pharmacologic treatments.
- Remove offending agents if possible.
- Iron replacement if low ferritin.
- Dopamine agonists, such as pramipexole and ropinirole, and benzodiazepines are first-line treatments.
- Gabapentin, gabapentin enacarbil (prodrug to gabapentin), and pregablin are also used.
- Low-potency opioids can be used for treatment-refractory patients.

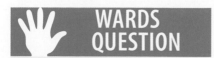

Q: What laboratory test should be ordered in a person diagnosed with Restless legs syndrome (RLS)? **A:** Serum ferritin.

SUBSTANCE/MEDICATION-INDUCED SLEEP DISORDER

- Severe sleep disorder due to substance intoxication/withdrawal or medication.
- Sleep disturbance not better explained by another sleep disorder (e.g., symptoms do not last longer than 1 month after intoxication or withdrawal).
- Can be insomnia, daytime sleepiness, parasomnia, or mixed type.
- Treatment is to remove the offending substance, or reduce, discontinue, or switch medications (if clinically appropriate).

NOTES

CHAPTER 16

SEXUAL DYSFUNCTIONS AND PARAPHILIC DISORDERS

Sexual dysfunctions include clinically significant disturbances in individuals' ability to respond sexually or to experience sexual pleasure.

Sexual Response Cycle

There are several stages of normal sexual response in men and women:

1. **Desire:** The motivation or interest in sexual activity, often reflected by sexual fantasies.
2. **Excitement/Arousal:** Begins with either fantasy or physical contact. It is characterized by erections and testicular enlargement in men and by vaginal lubrication, clitoral erection, labial swelling, and elevation of the uterus in the pelvis (*tenting*) in women. Both men and women experience flushing, nipple erection, and increased respiration, pulse, and blood pressure.
3. **Orgasm:** In men just prior there is tightening of the scrotal sac and secretion of a few drops of seminal fluid. Women experience contraction of the outer one-third of the vagina and enlargement of the upper one-third of the vagina.

   Men ejaculate and women have contractions of the uterus and lower one-third of the vagina. There is facial grimacing, release of tension, slight clouding of consciousness, involuntary anal sphincter contractions, and acute increase in blood pressure and pulse in both men and women.
4. **Resolution:** Muscles relax and cardiovascular state returns to baseline. Detumescence of genitalia in both sexes. Men have a *refractory period* lasting minutes to hours during which they cannot reexperience orgasm; women have little or no refractory period.

Sexual Changes with Aging

The desire for sexual activity does not usually change as people age. However, men usually require more direct stimulation of genitals and more time to achieve orgasm, with less reliable/strong erections. The intensity of ejaculation usually decreases, and the length of refractory period increases.

After menopause, women experience vaginal dryness and thinning due to decreased levels of estrogen and lubrication. They may also have decreased libido and reduced nipple/clitoral/vulvar sensitivity. These conditions can be treated with hormone replacement therapy or vaginal creams.

WARDS QUESTION

Q: Which class of antidepressants is most likely to cause sexual dysfunction?

A: Selective serotonin reuptake inhibitors (SSRIs).

Differential Diagnosis of Sexual Dysfunctions

Problems with sexual functioning may be due to any of the following:

- Medical conditions: Examples include atherosclerosis (causing erectile dysfunction from vascular occlusion), diabetes (causing erectile dysfunction from vascular changes and peripheral neuropathy), and pelvic adhesions (causing dyspareunia in women).
- Medication side effects: Antihypertensives, anticholinergics, antidepressants (especially selective serotonin reuptake inhibitors [SSRIs]), and antipsychotics.
- Depression.
- Substance use.

- Abnormal levels of gonadal hormones:
  - **Estrogen:** Decreased levels after menopause cause vaginal dryness and thinning in women (without affecting desire).
  - **Testosterone:** Promotes libido (desire) in both men and women.
  - **Progesterone:** May inhibit libido in both men and women by blocking androgen receptors; found in oral contraceptives, hormone replacement therapy, and, occasionally, treatments for prostate cancer.
- Presence of a sexual dysfunction (see below).

Sexual Dysfunctions

Sexual dysfunctions are problems involving any stage of the sexual response cycle. They all share the following *Diagnostic and Statistical Manual of Mental Disorders*, 5th ed. (*DSM-5*) criteria:

- The disorder causes clinically significant distress.
- The dysfunction is not better explained by a nonsexual mental disorder, as a consequence of severe relationship distress or other stressors, and not attributable to the effects of a substance/medication or another medical condition.

 Mr. Jones is a 58-year-old married man with a history of major depressive disorder who arrives at your outpatient clinic for a yearly follow-up visit. He complains of recent marital problems with his wife of 30 years. He is being treated with an SSRI, and his depressive symptoms have been stable for over 3 years on his current dose. Upon further questioning, he reveals that he has been having sex with his wife less often than usual, only once or twice a month. He states that this is a marked decrease since his last visit with you. He feels that lately they have been arguing more and feels that their decrease in sexual activity has adversely affected their relationship. He also reports a mild decrease in his energy.

Mr. Jones denies having urges to masturbate in the times between sexual intercourse with his wife. He also denies having any affairs, laughing nervously while saying, "I can barely satisfy my own wife." He appears sad and states that he is beginning to feel "down" about this. When he does have sex, he reports that it is initiated by his wife, and he is initially reluctant to engage in sexual activity. However, once he does, he denies any problems with having or sustaining an erection and denies any difficulties in reaching orgasm. Mr. Jones reports that he drinks two or three drinks per day on the weekends, and he does not use any recreational drugs.

What is his most likely diagnosis? What other considerations should be made?

The patient's most likely diagnosis is male hypoactive sexual desire disorder. Although decreased sexual interest is more prevalent in women, it should not be overlooked in men. As this clinical case shows, the patient does not seem to fantasize or desire sexual activity despite prior history of doing so. He appears distressed by this and reports that it is causing interpersonal dysfunction. Although his depression has remained stable during the past 3 years and the patient does not report symptoms that would suggest a current depressive episode, his sexual complaints and fatigue symptoms might suggest a relapse of depressive symptoms and should be monitored closely. It is also very important to consider if his treatment with an SSRI is affecting his sexual functioning.

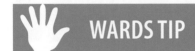

KEY FACT

Dopamine enhances libido. Serotonin inhibits sexual function.

WARDS TIP

Causes of sexual dysfunctions may be physiological, psychological, or both. Psychological causes of sexual dysfunctions are often comorbid with other psychiatric disorders, such as depression or anxiety.

WARDS TIP

Problems with sexual desire may be due to stress, relationship difficulties or conflict, poor self-esteem, or unconscious fears about sex.

> **What should you consider in the initial management of this patient's complaints?**
>
> His initial management should consist of a thorough history, a physical examination, and laboratory tests (complete metabolic profile, testosterone levels, thyroid-stimulating hormone levels) that might rule out medical (e.g., endocrine) abnormalities. If another medical disorder, mental disorder, or substance is not believed to be responsible, treatment considerations should include outpatient psychotherapy, sex therapy, cognitive-behavioral therapy, or group therapy.

WARDS QUESTION

Q: What are the most common sexual dysfunctions in men?
A: Erectile disorder and premature ejaculation.

KEY FACT

Other *DSM-5* categories of sexual dysfunction include substance/medication-induced sexual dysfunction and other specified/unspecified sexual dysfunction.

- **Male hypoactive sexual desire disorder:** Absence or deficiency of sexual thoughts, desire, or fantasies for more than 6 months (self-reported in approximately 5% of men).

- **Female sexual interest/Arousal disorder:** Absence or reduced sexual interest, thoughts/fantasies, initiation of sex, sexual excitement/pleasure, sexual arousal, and/or genital/nongenital sensations during sex for more than 6 months (unclear prevalence of *DSM-5* disorder, but self-reported in 26–43% of women).

- **Erectile disorder:** Marked difficulty obtaining or maintaining an erection, or marked decreased in erectile rigidity for more than 6 months. Commonly referred to as *erectile dysfunction (ED)* or *impotence*. May be *lifelong* (always had difficulty) or *acquired* (after previous ability to maintain erections). ED is the most common sexual disorder diagnosed in men; the prevalence is age dependent, from 5% at age 40 to 15% at age 70.

- **Premature (early) ejaculation:** Recurrent pattern of ejaculation during sex within 1 minute and before the individual wishes it for more than 6 months. Likely the most common sexual disorder in men, but underreported. Worldwide prevalence up to 30%.

- **Female orgasmic disorder:** Marked delay in infrequency/absence/reduced intensity of orgasm for more than 6 months. The international prevalence ranges from 20% to 40%.

- **Delayed ejaculation:** Marked delay in infrequency/absence of ejaculation for more than 6 months. Worse as men age and likely underreported, approximately 6% of men over 50 years report ejaculatory difficulty.

- **Genito-pelvic pain/Penetration disorder:** Persistent or recurrent difficulties in one of the following: vaginal penetration during intercourse, marked vulvovaginal or pelvic pain during intercourse or penetration, marked anticipatory fear or anxiety about vulvovaginal or pelvic pain, or marked tensing or tightening of pelvic floor muscles during attempted vaginal penetration for more than 6 months. Prevalence unknown but 10–20% of American women complain of pain during intercourse. Prior sexual/physical abuse is considered to be a risk factor.

Treatment of Sexual Disorders

SEX THERAPY

Sex therapy utilizes the concept of the couple, rather than the individual, as the target of therapy. Couples meet with a therapist together in sessions to identify and discuss their sexual problems. The therapist recommends sexual exercises for the couple to attempt at home; activities initially focus on heightening sensory awareness (sensate focus exercises) and progressively incorporate increased levels of sexual contact. Treatment is short term. This therapy is most useful when no other psychopathology is involved.

COGNITIVE-BEHAVIORAL THERAPY

Cognitive-behavioral therapy (CBT) approaches sexual dysfunction as a learned maladaptive behavior. It utilizes traditional therapies such as cognitive restructuring, partner communication training, systematic desensitization, and exposure, where patients are progressively exposed to increasing levels of stimuli that provoke their anxiety. Eventually, patients are able to respond appropriately to the stimuli. Other forms of therapy may include muscle relaxation techniques, assertiveness training, and prescribed sexual exercises to try at home. It is also a short-term therapy.

GROUP THERAPY

May be used as a primary or adjunctive therapy.

ANALYTICALLY ORIENTED (PSYCHODYNAMIC) PSYCHOTHERAPY

Individual, long-term therapy that focuses on feelings, past relationships (including familial), fears, fantasies, dreams, and interpersonal problems that may be contributing to the sexual disorder.

PHARMACOLOGIC TREATMENT

- **Erectile disorder:** Phosphodiesterase-5 inhibitors (e.g., sildenafil) are given orally, which enhance blood flow to the penis; they require psychological or physical stimulation to achieve an erection. A second-line treatment is alprostadil, either injected into the corpora cavernosa or transurethral, which acts locally; it produces an erection within 2–3 minutes and works in the absence of sexual stimulation.
- **Premature ejaculation:** SSRIs and the serotonergic tricyclic antidepressant (TCA) clomipramine prolong the time from stimulation to orgasm. Topical aesthetics are also occasionally used.
- **Male hypoactive sexual desire disorder/female sexual interest/arousal disorder:** Testosterone is used as replacement therapy for men with low levels. Low doses may also improve libido in women, especially in postmenopausal women. Medications that increase dopamine and norepinephrine, such as Flibanserin and bupropion, may also be used. Low-dose vaginal estrogen replacement may improve vaginal dryness and atrophy in postmenopausal women.

MECHANICAL THERAPIES

- **Erectile disorder:** Vacuum-assisted erection devices, penile prostheses, or surgical insertion of semirigid or inflatable tubes into the corpora cavernosa (used only for end-stage impotence).
- **Female orgasmic disorder:** Directed masturbation (education and self-awareness exercises to reach orgasm through self-stimulation).

- **Premature ejaculation:**
  - The *squeeze technique* is used to increase the threshold of excitability. When the man is excited to near ejaculation, he or his sexual partner is instructed to squeeze the glans of his penis in order to prevent ejaculation. Gradually, he gains awareness about his sexual sensations and learns to achieve greater ejaculatory control.
  - The *stop-start technique* involves cessation of all penile stimulation when the man is near ejaculation. This technique functions in the same manner as the squeeze technique.
- **Genito-pelvic pain/Penetration disorder:** Gradual desensitization to achieve intercourse, starting with muscle relaxation techniques, progressing to erotic massage, and finally achieving sexual intercourse.

Gender Dysphoria

Previous versions of the DSM included the diagnosis of *gender identity disorder*. This was revised to *gender dysphoria* in *DSM-5* to emphasize that the pathology is not gender diversity itself, but rather the **distress** caused by incongruence between the gender a person was assigned at birth and their identified gender.

Gender-expansive people experience disproportionately high rates of harassment, violence, and discrimination. One-third of transgender adults have had negative experiences related to their gender in healthcare settings, and nearly one-third are not "out" to any of their medical providers; therefore, clinicians should ask, not assume, a patient's gender, and use the patient's identified pronouns in all communication and documentation.

Common psychiatric comorbidities include suicidal ideation, mood/anxiety disorders, PTSD, substance use, and eating disorders.

DIAGNOSIS AND *DSM-5* CRITERIA

- **At least two of the following:**
  - A marked incongruence between one's experienced gender and primary/secondary sex characteristics.
  - A strong desire to be rid of one's primary/secondary sex characteristics because of the above.
  - A strong desire for the primary/secondary sex characteristics of the other gender.
  - A strong desire to be of the other gender.
  - A strong desire to be treated as the other gender.
  - A strong conviction that one has the typical feelings/reactions of the other gender.
- Clinically significant distress or impairment in functioning.

TREATMENT

Gender-affirming psychotherapy, and engagement of family support especially for children or adolescents. Transitioning may be social (e.g., changes to name, clothing, or hairstyle), medical (hormone therapy), or surgical. Surgical sex reassignment surgery can be performed after living 1 year in the desired gender role and 1 year of continuous hormone therapy. It's essential to screen carefully for comorbid psychiatric conditions and treat these as usual.

KEY FACT

Gender-expansive patients may use a wide range of terms to self-identify, such as transgender, nonbinary, or genderqueer. Transitioning is different for every individual, and may involve psychosocial changes, medications, or gender-affirming surgeries.

Paraphilias

Paraphilic disorders are characterized by engagement in unusual sexual activities and/or preoccupation with unusual sexual urges or fantasies for at least 6 months that either are acted on with a nonconsenting person or cause significant distress or impairment in functioning. Paraphilic fantasies alone are not considered disorders unless they are intense, recurrent, and interfere with daily life; occasional fantasies are considered normal components of sexuality (even if unusual).

Only a small percentage of people suffer from paraphilic disorders. Most paraphilic disorders occur almost exclusively in men, but sadism, masochism, and pedophilia may also occur in women. Voyeuristic and pedophilic disorders are the most common paraphilic disorders.

EXAMPLES OF PARAPHILIC DISORDERS

- **Pedophilic disorder:** Sexual fantasies/urges/behaviors involving sexual acts with prepubescent children (age 13 years or younger). *DSM-5* specifies that the person is at least age 16 and at least 5 years older than the child.
- **Frotteuristic disorder:** Sexual arousal from touching or rubbing against a nonconsenting person.
- **Voyeuristic disorder:** Sexual arousal from observing an unsuspecting nude, or disrobing individual (often with binoculars).
- **Exhibitionistic disorder:** Sexual arousal from exposure of one's genitals to an unsuspecting person.
- **Sexual masochism disorder:** Sexual arousal from the act of being humiliated, beaten, bound, or made to suffer.
- **Sexual sadism disorder:** Sexual arousal from the physical or psychological suffering of another person.
- **Fetishistic disorder:** Sexual arousal from either the use of nonliving objects (e.g., shoes or pantyhose) or nongenital body parts.
- **Transvestic disorder:** Sexual arousal from cross-dressing (e.g., man wearing women's clothing such as underwear).

COURSE AND PROGNOSIS

- *Poor prognostic factors* are having multiple paraphilias, early age of onset, comorbid substance use, high frequency of behavior, and referral by law enforcement agencies (i.e., after an arrest).
- *Good prognostic factors* are having only one paraphilia, self-referral for treatment, sense of guilt associated with the behavior, and history of otherwise normal sexual activity in addition to the paraphilia.

TREATMENT

- Difficult to treat; studied mostly in pedophilia.
- Psychotropic medication if associated with a comorbid psychiatric illness.

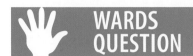

WARDS QUESTION

Q: What are the three most common types of paraphilia?
A: Pedophilia, voyeurism, and exhibitionism.

KEY FACT

Patients often have more than one paraphilia.

KEY FACT

An example of fetishistic disorder is a man being primarily sexually aroused by women's shoes resulting in significant distress and marital problems.

KEY FACT

An example of transvestic disorder is a person significantly distressed by being sexually aroused when dressing up as a member of the opposite gender. This is not the same as homosexuality or gender dysphoria.

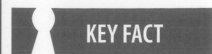

KEY FACT

Rape is a violent crime and not a paraphilia.

- Although controversial, antiandrogens, long-acting gonadotropin-releasing hormones, SSRIs, and naltrexone have been used to decrease sex drive and fantasies.
- Cognitive-behavioral therapy can be used to disrupt learned patterns and modify behavior.
- Social skills training.
- Twelve-step programs.
- Group therapy.

CHAPTER 17

PSYCHOTHERAPIES

It is common to combine psychotherapy with medications. *Split treatment* describes the arrangement where a physician prescribes medication and someone else provides therapy. In these cases, the physician and therapist should regularly communicate regarding the patient's treatment.

Psychoanalysis and Related Therapies

Psychoanalysis and its related therapies are derived from Sigmund Freud's psychoanalytic theories of the mind. Freud proposed that behaviors, or symptoms, result from *unconscious* mental processes, including defense mechanisms and conflicts between one's ego, id, superego, and external reality. Since the time of Freud, many other psychoanalytic theories have been developed. Influential theorists have included Melanie Klein, Heinz Kohut, Michael Balint, Margaret Mahler, and others.

Examples of psychoanalytic therapies include the following:

- Psychoanalysis.
- Psychoanalytically oriented psychotherapy.
- Brief dynamic therapy.
- Interpersonal therapy.

Freud's Theories of the Mind

TOPOGRAPHIC THEORY

1. **Unconscious:** Includes repressed thoughts that are out of one's awareness; involves *primary process* thinking (primitive, pleasure-seeking urges with no regard to logic or time, prominent in children and psychosis). Thoughts and ideas may be repressed into the unconscious because they are embarrassing, shameful, or otherwise too painful.
2. **Preconscious:** Contains memories that are easy to bring into awareness, but not unless consciously retrieved.
3. **Conscious:** Involves current thoughts and secondary process thinking (logical, organized, mature, and can delay gratification).

STRUCTURAL THEORY

1. **Id:** Unconscious; involves instinctual sexual/aggressive urges and primary process thinking.
2. **Superego:** Moral conscience and ego ideal (inner image of oneself that one wants to become).
3. **Ego:** Serves as a mediator between the id, superego, and external environment, and seeks to develop satisfying interpersonal relationships; uses *defense mechanisms* (see below) to control instinctual urges and distinguishes fantasy from reality using *reality testing*. Problems with reality testing occur in psychotic individuals.

Defense Mechanisms

Defense mechanisms are used by the ego to protect oneself and relieve anxiety by keeping conflicts out of awareness. They are (mostly) *unconscious* processes that are normal and healthy if they are mature and used in moderation (i.e.,

KEY FACT

Normal development: Id is present at birth, ego develops after birth, and superego development is traditionally considered to be completed by age 6.

KEY FACT

According to Freud, the superego is the aspect of one's psyche that represents "morality, society, and parental teaching."

KEY FACT

The Freudian superego represents internalization of cultural rules.

adaptive). They may be unhealthy if immature (i.e., maladaptive). Immature defense mechanisms can be used excessively as seen in some psychiatric disorders.

Defense mechanisms are often classified hierarchically. **Mature** defense mechanisms are healthy and adaptive, and they are seen in high-functioning and healthy adults. **Neurotic** defenses are encountered in obsessive-compulsive patients, patients with other anxiety disorders, and adults under stress. **Immature** defenses are seen in children, adolescents, psychotic patients, and some nonpsychotic patients, such as those with severe personality disorders. They are the most primitive defense mechanisms.

MATURE DEFENSES

Mature ego defenses are commonly found in healthy, high-functioning adults. These defenses often help people integrate conflicting emotions and thoughts.

1. **Altruism:** Performing acts that benefit others so as to vicariously experience pleasure. (*Clinical example:* A patient's child recently died from ovarian cancer. As part of the grieving process, the patient donates money to help raise community awareness about the symptoms of ovarian cancer so other patients could potentially benefit from early intervention.)
2. **Humor:** Expressing (usually) unpleasant or uncomfortable feelings without causing discomfort to self or others. (*Clinical Example:* When talking about lifestyle modifications, a diabetic patient jokingly reports that they are exercising their arm muscles when they eat.)
3. **Sublimation:** Satisfying socially objectionable impulses in an acceptable manner (thus *channeling* them rather than *preventing* them). (*Clinical example:* Person with unconscious urges to physically control others becomes a prison guard.)
4. **Suppression:** Purposely ignoring an unacceptable impulse or emotion so as to diminish discomfort and accomplish a task. (*Clinical example:* Nurse who feels nauseated by an infected wound puts aside feelings of disgust to clean wound and provides necessary patient care.)

NEUROTIC DEFENSES

1. **Displacement:** Shifting emotions from an undesirable situation to one that is personally tolerable. (*Clinical example:* Student who is angry with their mother talks back to their teacher the next day and refuses to obey instructions.)
2. **Intellectualization:** Avoiding negative feelings by excessive use of intellectual functions and by focusing on irrelevant details. (*Clinical example:* Physician dying from colon cancer describes the pathophysiology of the disease in detail to their 12-year-old child.)
3. **Isolation of affect:** Unconsciously limiting the experience of feelings or emotions associated with a stressful life event so as to avoid anxiety. (*Clinical example:* Patient describes the recent death of their beloved spouse without emotion.)
4. **Rationalization:** Explanations of an event to justify outcomes or behaviors and to make them acceptable. (*Clinical example:* "My boss fired me today because they aren't meeting their quotas, not because I haven't done a good job.")
5. **Reaction formation:** Doing the opposite of an unacceptable impulse. (*Clinical example:* Patient who is attracted to their married coworker insults them.)

KEY FACT

Suppression, as a defense mechanism, is a *conscious* process that involves avoiding paying attention to a particular emotion.

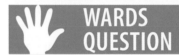

WARDS QUESTION

Q: A former gang member becomes a police officer working in the intercity to prevent gang violence. *What is the defense mechanism?*
A: Sublimation—The channeling of destructive impulses to create something constructive.

KEY FACT

Intellectualization is a defense mechanism where reasoning is used to block confrontation with an unconscious conflict or undesirable thought or feeling.

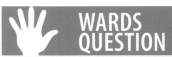

WARDS QUESTION

Q: An individual buys an unreasonably expensive new watch and tells their friends that they needed it because their old one was not reliable enough and they have to make sure to get to appointments on time. *What is the defense mechanism?*
A: Rationalization—Attempting to justify behavior to make it acceptable.

WARDS QUESTION

Q: A person accuses their partner of cheating when they themselves are involved in numerous affairs. *What is the defense mechanism?*
A: Projection—Ascribing one's objectional qualities onto others.

KEY FACT

Remember for individuals with borderline personality disorder, *splitting* is their major defense mechanism.

6. **Repression:** Preventing a thought or feeling from entering consciousness. (Repression is unconscious, whereas suppression is a conscious act.) (*Clinical Example:* A sexual assault victim tries hard but cannot recall details of the crime when questioned by police.)

IMMATURE DEFENSES

1. **Acting out:** Giving in to an impulse, even if socially inappropriate, so as to avoid the anxiety of suppressing that impulse. (*Clinical example:* Patient who has been told their therapist is going on vacation "forgets" their last appointment and skips it.)
2. **Denial:** Not accepting reality that is too painful. (*Clinical example:* Woman who has been scheduled for a breast mass biopsy cancels her appointment because she believes she is healthy.)
3. **Regression:** Performing behaviors from an earlier stage of development so as to avoid tension associated with current phase of development. (*Clinical example:* Patient brings their childhood teddy bear to the hospital when they have to spend the night.)
4. **Projection:** Attributing objectionable thoughts, qualities, or emotions to others. (*Clinical example:* An individual who is attracted to others believes their partner is having an affair.)

OTHER DEFENSE MECHANISMS

1. **Splitting:** Labeling people as all good or all bad; often seen in borderline personality disorder. (*Clinical example:* Patient who tells their doctor, "You and the nurses are the only people who understand me; all the other doctors are mean and impatient.")
2. **Undoing:** Attempting to reverse a situation by adopting a new behavior. (*Clinical example:* An individual who has had a brief fantasy of killing their spouse by sabotaging their car, takes the car in for a complete checkup.)

Psychoanalysis

The goal of psychoanalysis is to resolve *unconscious conflicts* by bringing repressed experiences and feelings into awareness and integrating them into the patient's conscious experience. Psychoanalysis is therefore considered *insight oriented*. Patients best suited for psychoanalysis have the following characteristics: not psychotic, intelligent, and stable in relationships and daily living. Treatment is usually 3–5 days per week for many years. During therapy sessions, the patient usually lies on a couch with the therapist seated out of view.

To become an analyst, professionals (MDs, PhDs, PsyDs, and MSWs) must complete training at a psychoanalytic institute. In addition to attending seminars and treating patients under supervision, the training requires that they receive their own analysis.

Psychoanalysis can be useful in the treatment of the following:
- Clusters B and C personality disorders.
- Anxiety disorders.
- Problems coping with life events.
- Sexual disorders.
- Persistent depressive disorder.

IMPORTANT CONCEPTS AND TECHNIQUES USED IN PSYCHOANALYSIS

- **Free association:** The patient is asked to say whatever comes into their mind during therapy sessions. The purpose is to bring forth thoughts and feelings from the unconscious so that the therapist may interpret them.
- **Dream interpretation:** Dreams are seen to represent conflict between urges and fears. Interpretation of dreams by the psychoanalyst is used to help achieve therapeutic goals.
- **Therapeutic alliance:** This is the bond between the therapist and the patient, who work together toward a therapeutic goal.
- **Transference:** Projection of unconscious feelings regarding important figures in the patient's life onto the therapist. Interpretation of transference is used to help the patient gain insight and resolve unconscious conflict.
- **Countertransference:** Projection of unconscious feelings about important figures in the therapist's life onto the patient. The therapist must remain aware of countertransference issues, as they may interfere with their objectivity.

PSYCHOANALYSIS-RELATED THERAPIES

Examples of psychoanalysis-related therapies include:

1. **Psychoanalytically oriented psychotherapy** and **brief dynamic psychotherapy:** These employ similar techniques and theories as psychoanalysis, but they are less frequent, less intense, usually briefer (weekly sessions for 6 months to several years), and involve face-to-face sessions between the therapist and patient (no couch).
2. **Interpersonal therapy:** Attachment-focused psychotherapy that centers on the development of skills to treat certain psychiatric disorders. Treatment is brief (once-weekly sessions for 3–4 months). The idea is to improve interpersonal relations. Sessions focus on reassurance, clarification of emotions, improving interpersonal communication, and testing perceptions. It has demonstrated efficacy in the treatment of depression and has been modified for use in adolescents.
3. **Supportive psychotherapy:** Purpose is to help patient feel safe during a difficult time and help to build up the patient's healthy defenses. Treatment is not insight oriented but instead focuses on empathy, understanding, and education. Supportive therapy is commonly used as adjunctive treatment in even the most severe mental disorders.

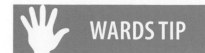

WARDS TIP

Psychoanalysis is not indicated for people who have problems with reality testing, such as actively psychotic or manic patients.

KEY FACT

An example of transference would be when a patient who has repressed feelings of abandonment by their parent becomes angry when their therapist is late for the appointment.

Behavioral Therapy

Behavioral therapy, pioneered by B. F. Skinner, seeks to treat psychiatric disorders by helping patients change behaviors that contribute to their symptoms. It can be used to extinguish maladaptive behaviors (such as phobic avoidance, compulsions, etc.) by replacing them with healthy alternatives. The time course is usually brief, and it is almost always combined with cognitive therapy as CBT.

LEARNING THEORY

Behavioral therapy is based on **learning theory**, which states that behaviors are learned by *conditioning* and can similarly be unlearned by *deconditioning*.

KEY FACT

Positive reinforcement: Giving a reward for a desired behavior.

KEY FACT

Negative reinforcement: Encouraging a behavior by removing an aversive stimulus. (*Example*: Putting on the seatbelt in the car to stop the beeping.) Punishment, in contrast, is an aversive response to a behavior. Punishment is *not* negative reinforcement.

KEY FACT

Biofeedback is used to treat a wide scope of clinical conditions including agoraphobia, fecal incontinence, tension headache, and hypertension.

CONDITIONING

- **Classical conditioning:** A neutral stimulus can evoke a conditioned response. (*Example:* Pavlov's dog would salivate when hearing a bell because the dog had learned that bells were always followed by food.)
- **Operant conditioning:** Behaviors can be learned when followed by positive or negative *reinforcement.* (*Example:* Skinner box—a rat presses a lever by accident and receives food; eventually, it learns to press the lever for food [trial-and-error learning].)

BEHAVIORAL THERAPY TECHNIQUES (DECONDITIONING)

- **Systematic desensitization:** The patient performs relaxation techniques while being exposed to increasing doses of an anxiety-provoking stimulus. Gradually, they learn to use relaxation skills to tolerate and cope with the anxiety-provoking stimulus. Commonly used to treat phobic disorders. (*Example:* A patient who has a fear of spiders is first shown a photograph of a spider, followed by exposure to a stuffed toy spider, then a videotape of a spider, and finally a live spider. At each step, the patient learns to relax while exposed to an increasing dose of the phobia.)
- **Flooding and implosion:** Through habituation, the patient is confronted with a real (flooding) or imagined (implosion) anxiety-provoking stimulus and not allowed to withdraw from it until they feel calm and in control. Relaxation exercises are used to help the patient tolerate the stimulus. Less commonly used than systematic desensitization to treat phobic disorders. (*Example:* A patient who has a fear of flying is made to fly in an airplane [flooding] or imagine flying [implosion].)
- **Aversion therapy:** A negative stimulus (such as an electric shock) is repeatedly paired with a specific behavior to create an unpleasant response. Used to treat addictions or paraphilic disorders. (*Example:* An alcoholic patient is prescribed Antabuse (disulfiram), which makes them ill every time they drink alcohol.)
- **Token economy:** Rewards are given after specific behaviors to positively reinforce them. Commonly used to encourage showering, shaving, and other positive behaviors in disorganized patients. Also frequently used in treatment of substance use disorders on rehabilitation units as part of a contingency management program where abstinence is reinforced with material rewards or privileges.
- **Biofeedback:** Physiological data (such as heart rate and blood pressure measurements) are given to patients as they try to mentally control physiological states. Can be used to treat anxiety disorders, migraines, hypertension, chronic pain, asthma, and incontinence. (*Example:* A patient is given their heart rate and blood pressure measurements during a migraine while being instructed to mentally control visceral changes that affect the pain.)

Cognitive Therapy

Cognitive therapy, pioneered by Aaron T. Beck, seeks to correct faulty assumptions and negative feelings that exacerbate psychiatric symptoms. The patient is taught to identify maladaptive thoughts and replace them with positive ones. It is most commonly used to treat depressive and anxiety disorders, and is usually combined with behavioral therapy in CBT. It may also be used for paranoid personality disorder, obsessive-compulsive disorder, somatic symptom disorders, and eating disorders. Cognitive therapy can be as effective as medication for some disorders.

CLINICAL EXAMPLE OF THE COGNITIVE THEORY OF DEPRESSION

- **Cognitive distortions**, also known as **faulty assumptions** or **automatic thoughts**. (*Example:* If I were smart, I would do well on tests. I must not be smart since I received average grades this semester.)
- **Negative thoughts.** (*Example:* I am stupid. I will never amount to anything worthwhile. Nobody likes a worthless person.)

Cognitive-Behavioral Therapy (CBT)

CBT combines theories and approaches from cognitive therapy and behavior therapy. Treatment follows a protocol or manual with homework assignments between therapy sessions. During therapy sessions, the patient and therapist set an **agenda**, review homework, and challenge cognitive distortions. The patients learn how their feelings and behavior are influenced by their thoughts. Treatment is usually brief and may last from 6 weeks to 6 months. Research has shown that CBT is effective for many psychiatric illnesses, including depression, anxiety disorders, schizophrenia, and substance use disorders.

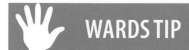

WARDS TIP

CBT focuses on a patient's current symptoms and problems by examining the connection between thoughts, feelings, and behaviors.

Mrs. R is a 22-year-old college student who is hospitalized after she tried to kill herself by taking an overdose of fluoxetine. This is her fifth overdose, and all have been in response to perceived rejections. She often feels "empty inside" and reports that she has had many intense relationships that have ended abruptly. She reports that she has been married for 1 year but fights constantly with her husband because of suspicions that he is unfaithful. Her husband denies these allegations and reports that he is tired of her outbursts, explaining that she yells at him and has become physically abusive. He has threatened to divorce her if these behaviors continue. During your evaluation, you notice multiple healed scars over her forearms, and she admits to self-harm behavior by cutting and burning herself because, "When I get angry, it helps me feel better."

During her hospitalization, you notice that her mood has improved and that she has become close to other patients. She says, "They are like family." Although you have seen her only twice, she thinks you are "a great doctor," unlike the psychiatrists who have treated her in the past, who have all been "idiots." You call her outpatient therapist, who confirms that she has been diagnosed with borderline personality disorder.

What are the recommended psychotherapeutic modalities for this patient?

Dialectical behavioral therapy (DBT) and psychoanalytic/psychodynamic therapy have shown to be effective treatments in randomized controlled trials for borderline personality disorder. DBT is a form of cognitive-behavioral therapy that is effective in reducing the urges to engage in self-harm behavior and leads to fewer hospital days. Although the efficacy of couples therapy in borderline patients has been debated, it might be considered in this case.

What special considerations should be taken into account when engaging in psychotherapy?

The psychotherapist should always be aware of positive or negative countertransference developed toward the patient. Frequent discussion and counseling with colleagues is useful. Patients with borderline personality disorder are challenging to treat due to their intense emotions, impulsivity, and anger.

What particular defense mechanism is exhibited by Mrs. R?

She exhibits splitting as evidenced by her extreme dichotomous thinking in expressing that you are a "great" psychiatrist, whereas other psychiatrists who have treated her in the past are "idiots."

Dialectical Behavioral Therapy (DBT)

DBT was developed by Marsha Linehan, and its effectiveness has been demonstrated in research trials. Once-weekly individual and group treatment can effectively diminish the self-destructive behaviors and hospitalizations of patients with borderline personality disorder. It incorporates cognitive and supportive techniques, along with "mindfulness" derived from traditional Buddhist practice. DBT has demonstrated effectiveness in patients with borderline personality disorders and eating disorders.

Group Therapy

- Three or more patients with a similar problem or pathology meet together with a therapist for group sessions. Many of the psychotherapeutic techniques already reviewed are used, including behavioral, cognitive, and supportive.

- Certain groups are *peer led* (including 12-step groups like Alcoholics Anonymous) and do not have a therapist present to facilitate the group. These groups meet to discuss problems, share feelings, and provide support to each other.

- Group therapy is especially useful in the treatment of substance use disorders, adjustment disorders, and personality disorders. Advantages of group therapy over individual therapy include:
  - Patients get immediate feedback and support from their peers.
  - Patients gain insight into their own condition by listening to others with similar problems.
  - If a therapist is present, there is an opportunity to observe interactions between others who may be eliciting a variety of transferences.

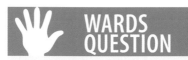

WARDS QUESTION

Q: What is the primary treatment for borderline personality disorder?

A: Dialectical behavioral therapy (DBT).

Family Therapy

Family therapy is useful as an adjunctive treatment in many psychiatric conditions because:

1. An individual's problems usually affect the entire family. They may be viewed differently and treated differently after the development of psychopathology, and new tensions and conflicts within the family may arise.

2. Psychopathology may arise or worsen due to dysfunction within the family unit. These conditions are most effectively treated with the entire family present. Evidence demonstrates that **high expressed emotion** (critical and

emotionally over-involved attitudes toward a family member) negatively impacts mental health in psychiatric patients.

The goals of family therapy are to reduce conflict, help members understand each other's needs (*mutual accommodation*), and help the family unit cope with internally destructive forces. **Boundaries** between family members may be too rigid or too permeable, and **"triangles"** may result when two family members form an alliance against a third member. The therapist may assist in correcting these problems. (*Example of boundaries that may be too permeable:* A parent and child smoke marijuana together and share intimate details about their sexual activities.) Family therapy is especially useful in treating schizophrenia and anorexia in adolescents.

Couples Therapy

Couples therapy is useful in the treatment of conflicts, sexual problems, and communication problems within the context of an intimate relationship. The therapist sees the couple together (**conjoint therapy**), but they may also be seen separately (**concurrent therapy**). In addition, each person may have a separate therapist and be seen individually (**collaborative therapy**). In the treatment of sexual problems, two therapists may see the couple together (**four-way therapy**). Relative contraindications include lack of motivation by one or both spouses and severe illness in one of the spouses (e.g., schizophrenia).

NOTES

CHAPTER 18

PSYCHOPHARMACOLOGY

Side Effects in a Nutshell

1. **HAM side effects** (*antiHistamine*—sedation, weight gain; *antiAdrenergic*—hypotension; *antiMuscarinic (anticholinergic)*—dry mouth, blurred vision, urinary retention, constipation, exacerbation of neurocognitive disorders (i.e., dementias).

   - Found in tricyclic antidepressants (TCAs) and low-potency antipsychotics.
   - Associated with increased risk of falls and delirium in elderly patients.

2. **Serotonin syndrome:** Confusion, flushing, diaphoresis, tremor, myoclonic jerks, hyperthermia, hypertonicity, rhabdomyolysis, renal failure, and death.

   - This uncommon psychiatric emergency occurs when there is too much serotonin, classically when selective serotonin reuptake inhibitors (SSRIs) and monoamine oxidase inhibitors (MAOIs) are combined. As this combination is rarely seen in practice anymore, serotonin syndrome is more commonly seen when a patient is prescribed multiple medications with serotonergic activity (e.g., SSRIs/SNRIs, lithium, trazodone, linezolid, Tramadol, triptans, dextromethorphan, St. John's wort, ondansetron), or other illicit drugs with serotonergic activity (e.g., cocaine, MDMA, amphetamine).
   - Treatment: Stop medications, supportive care, possibly use cyproheptadine or even ECT.

3. **Hypertensive crisis:** Caused by a buildup of stored catecholamines (norepinephrine); triggered by the combination of MAOIs with tyramine-rich foods (e.g., red wine, cheese, chicken liver, cured meats) or with sympathomimetics. Treated with IV phentolamine or sublingual nifedipine.

4. **Extrapyramidal side effects (EPS):** *Parkinsonism*—mask-like face, cogwheel rigidity, bradykinesia, pill-rolling tremor; *akathisia*—restlessness, need to move, and agitation; *dystonia*—sustained, painful contraction of muscles of neck, tongue, eyes, diaphragm.

   - Occur more frequently with high-potency, typical (first generation) antipsychotics, but can also be seen with atypical (second generation) antipsychotics.
   - Reversible.
   - All EPS can be treated with benztropine (Cogentin), although for akathisia, beta-blockers such as propranolol are first-line.
   - Occur within *hours to days* of starting medications or increasing doses.
   - In rare cases, can be life threatening (e.g., dystonia of the diaphragm causing asphyxiation).
   - Drug-induced parkinsonism should be differentiated from primary neurodegenerative Parkinson disease.

5. **Hyperprolactinemia:** Occurs with high-potency, typical (first generation) antipsychotics and risperidone.

6. **Tardive dyskinesia (TD):** Choreoathetoid (involuntary, irregular, and repetitive) muscle movements, usually of the mouth and tongue (can affect extremities, as well).

   - Occurs after *years* of antipsychotic use (more likely with high-potency, first-generation antipsychotics).
   - Usually irreversible.

7. **Neuroleptic malignant syndrome:** Mental status changes, fever, tachycardia, hypertension, tremor, hyporeflexia, elevated creatine phosphokinase (CPK), **"lead pipe" rigidity**.

   - Can be caused by any antipsychotic after a short or long time (increased with high-potency, typical antipsychotics).

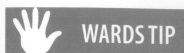

WARDS TIP

Drugs that increase serotonin may be found in over-the-counter medicines (e.g., dextromethorphan, St. John's wort). They can cause serotonin syndrome when taken in high doses or in combination with other serotonergic agents.

KEY FACT

Keeping the "kinesias" (impairment of body function) straight:

- Tardive dyskinesia is characterized by potentially permanent choreoathetoid movements and tongue protrusion.
- Acute dystonia is characterized by (painful and reversible) twisting and abnormal postures.
- Akathisia is characterized by the inability to sit still; feels like "ants in the pants."
- Bradykinesia is characterized by decreased or slow body movement.

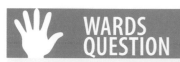

WARDS QUESTION

Q: What are the key differences between serotonin syndrome and neuroleptic malignant syndrome (NMS)?

A: Serotonin syndrome includes myoclonic jerks, hyperreflexia, hyperactive bowels, while NMS is marked by "lead pipe" rigidity, hyporeflexia, and ↑ CPK.

- A medical emergency with up to a 20% mortality rate.
- Treatment includes dantroline, bromocriptine, and ECT in emergencies.

8. **Drug interactions:** *Cytochrome P450* is a group of enzymes in the liver that metabolizes many common drugs, including psychiatric medications.

- Some medications *induce* the system, in other words the system metabolizes medications faster—drug levels *decrease.*
- Some medications *inhibit* the system, in other words the system metabolizes medications more slowly—drug levels *increase.*
- Common cytochrome P450 enzymes important in metabolizing psychiatric medications include CYP3A4, CYP2D6, CYP1A2, CYP2C9, and CYP2C19.
- For example: A patient with schizophrenia who smokes a pack of cigarettes a day is prescribed olanzapine. The tobacco *induces* CYP450 enzyme to metabolize the olanzapine quickly, the **d**rug level of olanzapine decreases, and the patient therefore requires a higher dose.

CYP450 *InDucers*	CYP450 *Inhibitors*
Tobacco (1A2)	Fluoxetine (2C19, 2C9, 2D6)
Carbamazepine (1A2, 2C9, 3A4)	Fluvoxamine (1A2, 2C19, 3A4)
Barbiturates (2C9)	Paroxetine (2D6)
St. John's wort (2C19, 3A4)	Sertraline (2D6)
	Duloxetine (2D6)

9. **Metabolic syndrome:** Antipsychotic medications (especially second-generation antipsychotics such as clozapine, olanzapine, quetiapine) can cause a metabolic syndrome which includes weight gain, hyperlipidemia, hyperglycemia, and hypertension that are associated with increased cardiovascular morbidity and mortality. Routine monitoring of patients on these medications should include weight checks or BMI, fasting lipid profile, A1C or fasting glucose, and vital signs; treatment with metformin may be considered.

Antidepressants

- The major categories of antidepressants are:
  - SSRIs.
  - SNRIs.
  - Heterocyclic antidepressants, including TCAs and tetracyclic antidepressants.
  - MAOIs.
  - Miscellaneous antidepressants.
- All antidepressants have similar response rates in treating major depression but differ in safety and side-effect profiles.
- Approximately 60–70% of patients with major depression will respond to an antidepressant medication.
- It usually takes 4–6 weeks on a given dose of an antidepressant for a patient to fully benefit from a trial of the medication, although many patients start responding sooner.
- For patients who are prone to side effects, it's important to start at a low dose and titrate up slowly.
- Some antidepressants have a *withdrawal phenomenon,* characterized by dizziness, headaches, nausea, insomnia, anxiety, electric-like shocks ("zaps"),

and malaise; depending on the dose and half-life, they may need to be tapered slowly before discontinuing.

- Because of their safety and tolerability, SSRIs and related antidepressants have become the most common agents used to treat major depression. However, the choice of a particular medication used for a given patient should be made based on:
  - Patient's particular symptoms
  - Previous treatment responses by the patient or a family member to a particular medication
  - Side-effect profile
  - Comorbid (medical and psychiatric) conditions
  - Risk of suicide via overdose on the medication
  - Cost (newer medications may be prohibitively expensive)

SELECTIVE SEROTONIN REUPTAKE INHIBITORS

- SSRIs inhibit presynaptic serotonin reuptake pumps, leading to increased availability of serotonin in synaptic clefts. Additionally, SSRIs cause downstream effects increasing brain plasticity—this mechanism has been hypothesized to explain the delay to onset of antidepressant effect.
- Although structural differences are minimal, patients often respond differently (in regards to efficacy and side effects) to different SSRIs.
- Based on their half-lives, most SSRIs can be dosed daily. Fluoxetine has a weekly dosing form available, as well.
- There is no correlation between plasma levels and efficacy or side effects.
- SSRIs are the most commonly prescribed antidepressants due to several distinct advantages:
  - Low incidence of side effects, most of which resolve with time.
  - No food restrictions.
  - Much safer in overdose.
- Examples of SSRIs include:
  - **Fluoxetine (Prozac):**
    - Longest half-life, with active metabolites; therefore, no need to taper.
    - Safe in pregnancy, approved for use in children and adolescents.
    - Common side effects: Insomnia, anxiety, sexual dysfunction.
    - Can elevate levels of antipsychotics, leading to increased side effects.
  - **Sertraline (Zoloft):**
    - Higher risk for gastrointestinal (GI) disturbances.
    - Very few drug interactions.
    - Other common side effects: Insomnia, anxiety, sexual dysfunction.
  - **Paroxetine (Paxil):**
    - A potent inhibitor of CYP26, which can lead to several drug–drug interactions.
    - Common side effects: Anticholinergic effects (e.g., sedation, constipation, weight gain) and sexual dysfunction.
    - Short half-life leading to uncomfortable *withdrawal phenomena* if not taken consistently.

KEY FACT

First-generation antipsychotics (typicals) are more associated with EPS and second-generation antipsychotics (atypicals) are more associated with metabolic side effects.

KEY FACT

The Food and Drug Administration (FDA) has a black box warning for all SSRIs potentially increasing "suicidal thinking and behavior." This warning applies to children and young adults to age 25, but may be accurate for older adults as well. The absolute risk remains low and must be weighed against the risks of an untreated mood disorder.

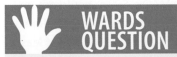

WARDS QUESTION

Q: How are sexual side effects of SSRI treated?
A: Either reducing the dose (if clinically appropriate), changing to a non-SSRI antidepressant, augmenting with bupropion, or, in men, by adding medications like sildenafil.

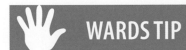

WARDS TIP

Patients should receive an adequate trial of antidepressant medication, usually at least 4–6 weeks at a full dose, before the medication is deemed non-efficacious.

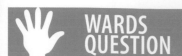

WARDS QUESTION

Q: What are the SSRIs associated with *most* and *least* weight gain? **A:** Paroxetine is the most associated with weight gain. Fluoxetine and sertraline are the most weight-neutral.

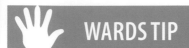

WARDS TIP

SSRIs can increase levels of warfarin, requiring increased monitoring when starting and stopping these medications.

KEY FACT

Serotonin syndrome is common when serotonergic drugs are used with MAOIs. SSRIs should not be used for at least 2 weeks before or after use of an MAOI, and at least 5–6 weeks with fluoxetine given its long half-life.

- **Fluvoxamine (Luvox):**
  - Currently approved only for use in obsessive-compulsive disorder (OCD).
  - Common side effects: Nausea and vomiting.
  - Multiple drug interactions due to CYP inhibition.
- **Citalopram (Celexa):**
  - Fewest drug–drug interactions.
  - Dose-dependent QTc prolongation.
- **Escitalopram (Lexapro):**
  - Levo-enantiomer of citalopram; similar efficacy, possibly fewer side effects.
  - Dose-dependent QTc prolongation.

Side Effects

- SSRIs have significantly fewer side effects than TCAs and MAOIs due to serotonin selectivity (not as much activity on histamine, adrenergic, or muscarinic receptors).
- They are much safer in overdose. Most side effects occur because of the extensive number of serotonin receptors throughout the body, including the GI tract.
- Many of the side effects of SSRIs resolve within a few days to weeks and include:
  - GI disturbance: Mostly nausea and diarrhea; giving with food can help.
  - Insomnia; also vivid dreams, often resolves over time.
  - Headache.
  - Weight changes (up or down).
- Other side effects include:
  - Sexual dysfunction (30–40%): Decreased libido, anorgasmia, delayed ejaculation. These may occur weeks to months after taking an SSRI and typically do not resolve.
  - Restlessness: An akathisia-like state.
  - **Serotonin syndrome:** Caused by an excess of serotonin in the body. It can result from taking a single serotonergic agent, or by taking multiple serotonergic agents in combination. One example is triptans (for migraine headaches) used with SSRIs. Serotonin syndrome is characterized by fever, diaphoresis, tachycardia, hypertension, delirium, and neuromuscular excitability (especially hyperreflexia and "electric jolt" limb movements), potentially death. Treatment includes stopping all serotonergic agents, administering cyproheptadine, and ECT in emergencies.
  - Hyponatremia: Rare.
  - Decreased platelet aggregation leading to increased risk of bleeding and bruising.
  - Seizures: Rate of approximately 0.2%, slightly lower than TCAs.

SEROTONIN-NOREPINEPHRINE REUPTAKE INHIBITORS (SNRIS)

- **Venlafaxine (Effexor):**
  - Often used for depressive disorders, anxiety disorders like generalized anxiety disorder (GAD), and neuropathic pain.

- Low drug interaction potential.
- Extended release (XR form) allows for once-daily dosing.
- Due to its short half-life, discontinuation of this drug should be tapered to avoid an uncomfortable discontinuation syndrome.
- Side-effect profile similar to SSRIs, with the exception of increased blood pressure (BP) in higher doses; do not use in patients with untreated or labile BP.
- New form, **desvenlafaxine (Pristiq)**, is the active metabolite of venlafaxine; it is expensive and without known benefit over venlafaxine.
- **Duloxetine (Cymbalta):**
  - Often used for people with **depression, neuropathic pain**, and in fibromyalgia.
  - Side effects are similar to SSRIs (no hypertensive risk), but more constipation relating to its norepinephrine effects.
  - Hepatotoxicity may be more likely in patients with liver disease or heavy alcohol use, so liver function tests should be monitored when indicated.

MISCELLANEOUS ANTIDEPRESSANTS

- **Bupropion (Wellbutrin):**
  - Norepinephrine-dopamine reuptake inhibitor.
  - Relative **lack of sexual side effects** as compared to the SSRIs. Can be added to other antidepressants to treat sexual dysfunction.
  - Some efficacy in treatment of adult attention deficit hyperactivity disorder (ADHD).
  - Effective for smoking cessation.
  - Weight neutral.
  - Side effects include increased anxiety, as well as increased risk of **seizures** and psychosis at high doses.
  - Contraindicated in patients with epilepsy or active eating disorders, and in those currently on an MAOI. Use with caution with agents that also lower the seizure threshold (like stimulants).

Serotonin Receptor Antagonists and Agonists

- **Trazodone (Desyrel)** and **Nefazodone (Serzone):**
  - Useful in the treatment of major depression, major depression with anxiety, and **insomnia** (secondary to its sedative effects).
  - They do not have the sexual side effects of SSRIs and do not affect rapid eye movement (REM) sleep.
  - Side effects include nausea, dizziness, orthostatic hypotension, cardiac arrhythmias, **sedation**, and **priapism** (especially with **trazodone**).
  - Because of orthostatic hypotension and sedation in higher doses, trazodone is not frequently used solely as an antidepressant. It is commonly used to treat insomnia often when initiating an SSRI (until insomnia improves as the depression resolves).
  - Nefazodone carries a **black box warning** for rare but serious liver failure (1 per 250,000–300,000 people) and is now off the market.

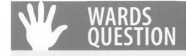

WARDS QUESTION

Q: Which antidepressant is least likely to cause sexual side effects? **A:** Wellbutrin (bupropion).

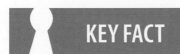

KEY FACT

Trazodone causes priapism: Remember the phrase "Trazo-bone."

α2-Adrenergic Receptor Antagonists

- **Mirtazapine (Remeron):**
  - Mechanism of action is antagonism of the central presynaptic alpha-2-adrenergic receptors, which causes an increased release of serotonin and norepinephrine.
  - Useful in the treatment of **major depression**, especially in patients who have significant weight loss and/or insomnia.
  - At lower doses, mirtazapine acts preferentially on histamine receptors causing sedation and increased appetite, but at higher doses acts preferentially on the norepinephrine receptors and can be more activating.
  - Side effects include **sedation**, **weight gain**, dizziness, tremor, dry mouth, constipation, and (rarely) agranulocytosis.
  - Fewer sexual side effects compared to SSRIs and few drug interactions.

HETEROCYCLIC ANTIDEPRESSANTS

- TCAs inhibit the reuptake of norepinephrine and serotonin, increasing availability of monoamines in the synapse.
- Because of the long half-lives, most are dosed once daily.
- They are rarely used as first-line agents due to a higher incidence of side effects, titration of dosing, and **lethality in overdose**.

TRICYCLIC ANTIDEPRESSANTS

- **Tertiary amines** (highly anticholinergic/antihistaminergic [more sedating]/ antiadrenergic [more orthostasis] with a greater lethality in overdose):
  - **Amitriptyline (Elavil):** Useful in chronic pain, migraines, and insomnia.
  - **Imipramine (Tofranil):**
    - Has intramuscular form.
    - Useful in **enuresis** and panic disorder.
  - **Clomipramine (Anafranil):** Most serotonin-specific, therefore has efficacy in the treatment of **OCD**.
  - **Doxepin (Sinequan):**
    - Useful in treating chronic pain.
    - Used as a sleep aid in low doses.
- **Secondary amines**—Metabolites of tertiary amines (less anticholinergic/ antihistaminic/antiadrenergic):
  - **Nortriptyline (Pamelor, Aventyl):**
    - Least likely to cause orthostatic hypotension.
    - Useful therapeutic blood levels.
    - Useful in treating chronic pain.
    - Can be safely used in geriatric population.
  - **Desipramine (Norpramin):**
    - More activating/least sedating.
    - Least anticholinergic.

KEY FACT

Mirtazapine (Remeron) is good for treating major depression in the elderly—It helps with both sleep and appetite.

TETRACYCLIC ANTIDEPRESSANTS

- **Amoxapine (Asendin):**
  - Metabolite of antipsychotic loxapine.
  - May cause EPS and has a similar side-effect profile to typical antipsychotics.

Side Effects

- TCAs are *highly* protein bound and lipid soluble, and therefore can interact with other medications that have high protein binding.
- The side effects of TCAs are mostly due to their lack of specificity and interaction with other receptors.
- Antihistaminic properties: Sedation and weight gain.
- Antiadrenergic properties (**cardiovascular** side effects): Orthostatic hypotension, dizziness, reflex tachycardia, arrhythmias (block cardiac sodium channel), and electrocardiographic (ECG) changes (widening QRS, QT, and PR intervals). Avoid in patients with preexisting conduction abnormalities or recent MI, or with increased fall risk.
- Antimuscarinic effects (also called anticholinergic): Dry mouth, constipation, urinary retention, blurred vision, tachycardia, and exacerbation of narrow angle glaucoma. Can lead to delirium in the elderly population.
- Lethal in overdose—Must carefully assess the suicide risk when prescribing. Symptoms of overdose include agitation, tremors, ataxia, arrhythmias, delirium, hypoventilation from central nervous system (CNS) depression, myoclonus, hyperreflexia, seizures, and coma.
- Seizures: Risk of seizure is directly related to the dose and serum level (i.e., higher risk of seizures at high doses and overdoses).
- Serotonergic effects: Erectile/ejaculatory dysfunction in males, anorgasmia in females.

MONOAMINE OXIDASE INHIBITORS

- MAOIs prevent the inactivation of biogenic amines such as *norepinephrine*, *serotonin*, *dopamine*, and *tyramine* (an intermediate in the conversion of tyrosine to norepinephrine).
- By **irreversibly** inhibiting the enzymes *MAO-A* and *B*, MAOIs increase the number of neurotransmitters available in synapses.
- MAO-A preferentially deactivates serotonin and norepinephrine, and MAO-B preferentially deactivates phenethylamine; *both* types also act on dopamine and tyramine.
- MAOIs are not used as first-line agents because of the increased safety and tolerability of newer agents, notably SSRIs/SNRIs. However, MAOIs are rarely used for certain types of **refractory depression** and in refractory anxiety disorders:
  - **Phenelzine (Nardil).**
  - **Tranylcypromine (Parnate).**
  - **Isocarboxazid (Marplan).**

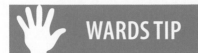

A 1-week supply of TCAs (as little as 1–2 g) can be **lethal** in overdose.

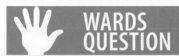

Q: What is the treatment for TCA overdose?
A: IV sodium bicarbonate.

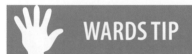

Major complications of TCAs—3Cs:
Cardiotoxicity
Convulsions
Coma

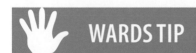

Q: What are the most common side effects of TCAs?
A: Anticholinergic effects: Dry mouth, urinary retention, constipation, and blurry vision.

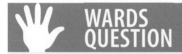

MAOIs are considered more effective than TCAs in depression with atypical features, characterized by hypersomnia, increased appetite, heavy feeling in extremities, and increased sensitivity to interpersonal rejection.

Side Effects

- **Serotonin syndrome** occurs when **SSRIs** and **MAOIs** are taken together or if other drugs cause increase in serotonin levels.
  - Initially characterized by lethargy, restlessness, confusion, flushing, hyperactive bowels, diaphoresis, tremor, and myoclonic jerks.
  - May progress to hyperthermia, hypertonicity, rhabdomyolysis, renal failure, convulsions, coma, and death.
  - Treatment includes immediately discontinuing serotonergic medications, ICU monitoring, and administration of cyproheptadine. ECT can be effective.
  - Wait at least 2 weeks before switching from SSRI to MAOI, and at least 5–6 weeks with fluoxetine.
- **Hypertensive crisis:** Risk when MAOIs are taken with tyramine-rich foods or sympathomimetics.
  - Foods with tyramine (red wine, cheese, chicken liver, fava beans, cured meats) cause a buildup of stored catecholamines.
  - In addition to a markedly elevated BP, it is also characterized by headache, sweating, nausea, and vomiting, photophobia, autonomic instability, chest pain, arrhythmias, and death.
- Orthostatic hypotension (most common).
- Drowsiness.
- Weight gain.
- Sexual dysfunction.
- Dry mouth.
- Sleep dysfunction.
- Patients with pyridoxine deficiency can have numbness or paresthesias, so they should supplement with B_6.
- Liver toxicity, seizures, and edema (rare).
- *"Start low and go slow"* (low doses that are increased slowly).

WARDS TIP

Selegiline (Emsam transdermal patch) is a MAOI used to treat depression that does not require following the dietary restrictions when used in low dosages. However, decongestants, opiates (such as meperidine, fentanyl, and tramadol), and serotonergic drugs must still be avoided.

Antidepressant Use in Other Disorders

- OCD: SSRIs (in high doses), TCAs (clomipramine).
- Panic disorder: SSRIs, SNRIs, TCAs, MAOIs.
- Eating disorders: SSRIs (in high doses), TCAs.
- Persistent depressive disorder (dysthymia): SSRIs, SNRIs (e.g., venlafaxine, duloxetine).
- Social anxiety disorder (social phobia): SSRIs, SNRIs, MAOIs.
- GAD: SSRIs, SNRIs (venlafaxine), TCAs.
- Posttraumatic stress disorder: SSRIs.
- Irritable bowel syndrome: SSRIs, TCAs.
- Enuresis: TCAs (imipramine).
- Neuropathic pain: TCAs (amitriptyline and nortriptyline), SNRIs.
- Chronic pain: SNRIs, TCAs.
- Fibromyalgia: SNRIs.
- Migraine headaches: TCAs (amitriptyline).

- Smoking cessation: Bupropion.
- Premenstrual dysphoric disorder: SSRIs.
- Insomnia: Mirtazapine, trazodone, TCAs (doxepin).

Antipsychotics

- Antipsychotics are used to treat psychotic disorders and bipolar disorders, as well as psychotic symptoms associated with other psychiatric and medical illnesses.
  - *Typical* or *first-generation* antipsychotics, sometimes referred to as neuroleptics, are classified according to potency and treat psychosis by primarily by blocking dopamine (D2) receptors.
  - *Atypical* or *second-generation* antipsychotics block both dopamine (D2) and serotonin (5HT-2A) receptors.
- Most antipsychotics have a number of actions and receptor interactions in the brain that contribute to their varied efficacy and side-effect profiles.
- Both typical and atypical antipsychotics have similar efficacies in treating the presence of *positive psychotic symptoms*, such as hallucinations and delusions.
- Atypical antipsychotics were thought to be more effective at treating *negative symptoms* (such as flattened affect and social withdrawal), although this has not been consistently shown in the literature.
- Atypical antipsychotics have largely replaced typical antipsychotics in use due to their side-effect profile. However, the risk of metabolic syndrome/ weight gain and other side effects, as well as the significant cost of the atypical antipsychotics means that currently both classes are used as first-line treatments.
- The choice of which specific medication to prescribe should be made based on the patient's individual clinical presentation, past response (favorable and unfavorable), side-effect profile, and preference.

TYPICAL (FIRST-GENERATION) ANTIPSYCHOTICS

All typical antipsychotics have similar efficacy, but vary in potency.

Low-Potency, Typical Antipsychotics

- Lower affinity for dopamine receptors and therefore a higher dose is required. Remember, *potency* refers to the action on dopamine receptors, *not* the level of efficacy.
- Higher incidence of antiadrenergic, anticholinergic, and antihistaminic side effects compared to high-potency typical antipsychotics.
- Lower incidence of EPS and (possibly) neuroleptic malignant syndrome.
- More lethality in overdose due to QTc prolongation, and the potential for heart block and ventricular tachycardia.
- Rare risk of agranulocytosis, and slightly higher seizure risk than high-potency antipsychotics.
  - **Chlorpromazine (Thorazine):**
    - Commonly causes orthostatic hypotension.
    - Can cause blue-gray skin discoloration as well as corneal and lens deposits.

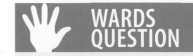

WARDS QUESTION

Q: How is serotonin syndrome treated?
A: First, discontinue the medication(s), next, provide supportive care and benzodiazepines. The serotonin antagonist cyproheptadine and ECT can also be used.

WARDS TIP

Warning about atypical antipsychotics: Although they are used to treat the behavioral symptoms of neurocognitive disorders (dementias) and delirium, studies show an increased risk of all-cause mortality and stroke when using these agents in the elderly, which, as a result, is listed as a FDA black box warning for these medications.

- Can lead to photosensitivity.
- Also used to treat nausea and vomiting, as well as intractable hiccups.
- Comes in PO and IM formulations (effective in treating agitation in emergencies).

- **Thioridazine (Mellaril):** Associated with retinitis pigmentosa.

Midpotency, Typical Antipsychotics

■ Have midrange properties.

- **Loxapine (Loxitane):**
  - Higher risk of seizures.
  - Metabolite is an antidepressant.
- **Thiothixene (Navane):** Can cause ocular pigment changes.
- **Molindone (Moban).**
- **Perphenazine (Trilafon).**

High-Potency, Typical Antipsychotics

■ Greater affinity for dopamine receptors; therefore, a relatively low dose is needed to achieve effect.

■ Less sedation, orthostatic hypotension, and anticholinergic effects.

■ Greater risk for extrapyramidal symptoms and (likely) TD.

- **Haloperidol (Haldol):** Can be given PO/IM/IV. Decanoate (long acting) form available.
- **Fluphenazine (Prolixin):** Can be given PO/IM. Decanoate form available.
- **Trifluoperazine (Stelazine):** Approved for nonpsychotic anxiety.
- **Pimozide (Orap):** Associated with QTc prolongation and ventricular tachycardia.

Ms. B is a 28-year-old, overweight female who presents to your outpatient clinic following discharge from an inpatient psychiatry unit. Police found her in a local shopping mall, talking to herself and telling a passerby that the devil had "stolen her soul." She appeared disheveled and scared. During the hospitalization, she was diagnosed with schizophrenia, and olanzapine was prescribed and titrated to 30 mg at bedtime for delusional thinking and disorganized behavior. She has since been living with her parents, and her hygiene and self-care have improved. Although Ms. B reports occasional auditory hallucinations telling her that her parents do not like her, she recognizes that the voices are not real and is not distressed by them. She has become involved in a vocational skills program and hopes to work at a local supermarket. However, during her last appointment with her primary care doctor, she was told she had an elevated fasting glucose of 115 and triglycerides of 180, and that she had gained 12 pounds in the past 3 months with a waist circumference of 36 inches. Her blood pressure was normal, but she reported a family history of diabetes and high blood pressure.

What is the next step?

Given her diagnosis of schizophrenia, and that Ms. B has had an adequate partial response to pharmacological treatment, she should continue to be treated with an antipsychotic. However, her recent laboratory results are suggestive of metabolic syndrome, and thus she is at an increased risk for cardiovascular disease. While this patient has responded well to olanzapine, this medication along with other atypical antipsychotics have been associated with increased weight gain and impaired glucose metabolism. It is unclear if her laboratory test results were abnormal prior to starting olanzapine, are elevated secondary to treatment, or a combination of both. In treating Ms. B, first steps include recommending lifestyle modifications and close monitoring of her weight, blood sugar levels, lipids, and waist circumference, while collaborating closely with her primary care physician. If a change in her antipsychotic medication is warranted after weighing the risks and benefits of altering her treatment, other atypical antipsychotics such as ziprasidone or aripiprazole (both less associated with weight gain), or typical antipsychotics might be considered; these medications would then be cross-tapered. When choosing medications, consideration must be given to a history of response, tolerability, side-effect profile, patient preference, and cost.

Side Effects

- The positive symptoms of schizophrenia are treated by action of the medications in the mesolimbic dopamine pathway. The mesolimbic pathway includes the nucleus accumbens, the fornix, the amygdala, and the hippocampus.
- The negative symptoms of schizophrenia are thought to occur due to (decreased) dopaminergic action in the mesocortical pathway.
- Extrapyramidal symptoms occur through blockade of the dopamine pathways in the nigrostriatum.
- Increased prolactin is caused by dopamine blockade in the tuberoinfundibular area.
- **Antidopaminergic effects:**
  - EPS:
    - *Parkinsonism*—Bradykinesia, mask-like face, cogwheel rigidity, pill-rolling tremor. Treat with benztropine (Cogentin) or lower dose if appropriate.
    - *Akathisia*—Subjective anxiety and restlessness, objective fidgetiness. Patients may report a sensation of inability to sit still. Best treated with dose reduction (if appropriate), β-blockers, or benzodiazepines.
    - *Dystonia*—Sustained painful contraction of muscles of neck (*torticollis*), tongue, eyes (*oculogyric crisis*). It can be life threatening if it involves the airway or diaphragm. Treat with benztropine (Cogentin) or diphenhydramine (Benadryl), or lower the dose if appropriate.
  - **Hyperprolactinemia**—Leads to decreased libido, galactorrhea, gynecomastia, impotence, amenorrhea.
- **Anti-HAM effects:** Caused by actions on **H**istaminic, **A**drenergic, and **M**uscarinic receptors:
  - *Antihistaminic*—Results in sedation, **weight gain**.
  - *Anti-α1 adrenergic*—Results in orthostatic hypotension, cardiac abnormalities, and sexual dysfunction.
  - *Antimuscarinic*—Anticholinergic effects, resulting in dry mouth, tachycardia, urinary retention, blurry vision, constipation, and precipitation of narrow-angle glaucoma.
- **Tardive dyskinesia:**
  - Choreoathetoid (writhing, irregular) movements of mouth and tongue (or other body parts) that may occur in patients who have used antipsychotics for more than 6 months.

KEY FACT

Haloperidol (Haldol) is often given as an intramuscular injection to treat acute agitation or psychosis. The commonly used phrase: "5 and 2," in psychiatric emergencies refers to 5 mg of IM haloperidol and 2 mg of IM lorazepam in order to quickly sedate an agitated patient.

WARDS TIP

Haloperidol and fluphenazine are also available in long-acting, intramuscular forms (decanoate) that are useful if patients are poorly compliant with their oral medication. Risperidone (Consta), aripiprazole (Maintena), and paliperidone (Invega Sustenna) also have long-acting injectibles, but they are more expensive.

KEY FACT

There is a roughly 5% chance of developing tardive dyskinesia for each year treated with a typical antipsychotic.

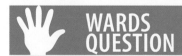

WARDS QUESTION

Q: How are dystonia and akathisia treated?
A: The first-line treatment for dystonia is benztropine (Cogentin). Diphenhydramine (Benadryl) can also be used. The first-line treatment for akathisia is decreasing the dose of the causative agent (if appropriate), or adding propranolol or a benzodiazepine.

KEY FACT

Clozapine, the first atypical antipsychotic, is less likely to cause tardive dyskinesia.

- Older age is a risk factor.
- Women and patients with affective disorders *may* be at an increased risk.
- Although up to 50% of cases will remit (without further antipsychotic use), most cases are *permanent*.
- Treatment involves discontinuation of current antipsychotic if clinically possible and changing to a medication with less potential to cause TD.

■ Less common side effects include **neuroleptic malignant syndrome (NMS)**:

- Though uncommon, occurs more often in *young males early in treatment* with *high-potency typical antipsychotics*.
- It is a **medical emergency** and has up to a 20% mortality rate if left untreated.
- It is characterized by **FALTERED**:
  - **F**ever (most common presenting symptom).
  - **A**utonomic instability (tachycardia, labile hypertension, diaphoresis).
  - **L**eukocytosis.
  - **T**remor.
  - **E**levated CPK.
  - **R**igidity (*lead pipe* rigidity is considered almost universal).
  - **E**xcessive sweating (diaphoresis).
  - **D**elirium (mental status changes).
- **Treatment** involves discontinuation of current medications and administration of supportive medical care (hydration, cooling, etc.).
- Sodium dantrolene, bromocriptine, and amantadine may be used but have their own side effects and unclear efficacy. ECT can also be effective.
- This is *not* an allergic reaction.
- Patient is not prevented from restarting the same antipsychotic at a later time, but will have an increased risk for another episode of neuroleptic malignant syndrome.

■ Elevated liver enzymes, jaundice.

■ **Ophthalmologic** problems (irreversible retinal pigmentation with high doses of thioridazine, deposits in lens and cornea with chlorpromazine).

■ **Dermatologic** problems, including rashes and photosensitivity (blue-gray skin discoloration with chlorpromazine).

■ **Seizures:** All antipsychotics lower the seizure threshold, although low-potency antipsychotics are more likely.

ATYPICAL (SECOND-GENERATION) ANTIPSYCHOTICS

■ Atypical antipsychotics block both dopamine and serotonin receptors and are associated with different side effects than typical antipsychotics.

■ In particular, they are less likely to cause EPS, TD, or neuroleptic malignant syndrome.

■ They *may* be more effective than typical antipsychotics in treating **negative symptoms** of schizophrenia.

■ Atypical antipsychotics are also used to treat acute mania, bipolar disorder, and as adjunctive medications in unipolar depression.

■ They are also used in treating borderline personality disorder, PTSD, and certain psychiatric disorders in childhood (e.g., tic disorders).

- **Clozapine (Clozaril):**
  - Less likely to cause TD.
  - Only antipsychotic shown to be **more efficacious** than the others; used in **treatment refractory schizophrenia.**
  - Only antipsychotic shown to decrease **the risk of suicide.**
  - More anticholinergic side effects than other atypical or high-potency typical antipsychotics. Associated with tachycardia, constipation, and hypersalivation.
  - **Risk of severe side effects**
    - 1% incidence of **agranulocytosis;** clozapine must be stopped if the *absolute neutrophil count (ANC)* drops below 1500 per microliter. All patients must undergo regular ANC monitoring weekly for the first 6 months of treatment, followed by biweekly for 6 months, and then monthly monitoring.
    - 4% incidence of **seizures.**
    - Small risk of **myocarditis.**
- **Risperidone (Risperdal):**
  - Can cause increased prolactin.
  - Associated with orthostatic hypotension and reflex tachycardia.
  - Long-acting injectable (LAI) form named Consta.
- **Quetiapine (Seroquel):** Much less likely to cause EPS; common side effects include sedation, orthostatic hypotension, and weight gain.
- **Olanzapine (Zyprexa):** Common side effects include significant weight gain, sedation, and dyslipidemia. Comes in PO/IM/LAI formulations.
- **Ziprasidone (Geodon):** Less likely to cause significant weight gain, associated with QTc prolongation, and must be taken with food (50% reduction in absorption without a 300-calorie meal). Comes in PO and IM formulations.
- **Aripiprazole (Abilify):**
  - Unique mechanism of partial D2 agonism.
  - Can be more activating (akathisia) and less sedating.
  - Less potential for weight gain.
  - Comes in PO, IM, and LAI formulations.
- Newer (more expensive) antipsychotics:
  - **Paliperidone (Invega):**
    - Metabolite of risperidone.
    - Long-acting injectable forms: Sustenna—monthly; Trinza—every 3 months.
  - **Asenapine (Saphris) orally dissolving (sublingual) tablet.**
  - **Iloperidone (Fanapt).**
  - **Lurasidone (Latuda): Must be taken with food; used in bipolar depression.**

Side Effects

- **Metabolic syndrome.**
  - This must be monitored with baseline weight, waist circumference (measured at iliac crest), BP, HbA1c, and fasting lipids.

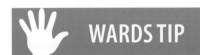

WARDS TIP

Onset of antipsychotic side effects
NMS: Any time (but usually early in treatment)
Acute dystonia: Hours to days
Parkinsonism/Akathisia: Days to weeks
Tardive dyskinesia: Months to years
The **Abnormal Involuntary Movement Scale (AIMS)** can be used to quantify and monitor for tardive dyskinesia.

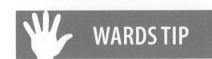

WARDS TIP

Thirty percent of patients with treatment-resistant psychosis will respond to clozapine.

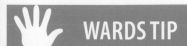

WARDS TIP

Patients on clozapine must have weekly blood draws for the first 6 months to check WBC and absolute neutrophil counts because of the risk of agranulocytosis. With time, the frequency of blood draws decreases.

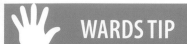

WARDS TIP

Quetiapine, olanzapine, aripiprazole, risperidone, asenapine, and ziprasidone have FDA approval for treatment of mania.

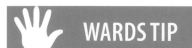

WARDS TIP

Antipsychotics may be used as adjuncts to mood stabilizers early in the course of a manic episode. Atypical antipsychotics are often prescribed as monotherapy in the acute or maintenance treatment of bipolar disorder.

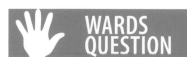

WARDS QUESTION

Q: What is the only mood stabilizer shown to decrease suicidality?
A: Lithium.

- **Weight gain:** Metformin can be used to reduce or prevent.
- Hyperlipidemia.
- Hyperglycemia—Rarely, **diabetic ketoacidosis** has been reported.

■ Some anti-HAM effects (antihistaminic, antiadrenergic, and antimuscarinic).

■ Elevated liver function tests (LFTs)—Monitor yearly for elevation in LFTs and ammonia.

■ QTc prolongation.

Mood Stabilizers

■ Mood stabilizers are used to treat **acute mania** and to help **prevent relapses** of manic episodes (maintenance treatment) in bipolar disorder and schizoaffective disorder. Less commonly, they may be used for:

- Augmentation of antidepressants in patients with major depression refractory to monotherapy.
- Potentiation of antipsychotics in patients with schizophrenia or schizoaffective disorder.
- Treatment of aggression and impulsivity (e.g., neurocognitive disorders, intellectual disability, personality disorders, other medical conditions).
- Enhancement of abstinence in treatment of alcoholism.

■ Mood stabilizers include lithium and anticonvulsants, most commonly valproic acid, lamotrigine, and carbamazepine.

LITHIUM

■ Lithium is the drug of choice in acute mania and as prophylaxis for both manic and depressive episodes in bipolar and schizoaffective disorders.

■ It is also used in cyclothymic disorder and unipolar depression.

■ Lithium is metabolized by the kidney, so dosing adjustments may be necessary in patients with renal dysfunction.

■ Prior to initiating, patients should have an ECG, basic chemistries, thyroid function tests, a complete blood count (CBC), and a pregnancy test.

■ Onset of action takes 5–7 days.

■ Blood levels correlate with clinical efficacy and should be checked 4–5 days after initiation of treatment and after every dose change.

■ The major drawback of lithium is its high incidence of side effects and very narrow therapeutic index:

- Therapeutic range: 0.6–1.2. (Individual patients can have significant side effects even within this range.)
- Toxic: >1.5.
- Potentially lethal: >2.0.

Side Effects

■ Toxic levels of lithium cause altered mental status, coarse tremors, convulsions, delirium, coma, and death.

■ Clinicians need to regularly monitor blood levels of lithium, thyroid function (thyroid-stimulating hormone), and kidney function.

- Fine tremor.
- Cognitive slowing or dulling.
- Nephrogenic diabetes insipidus (polydipsia, polyuria).
- GI disturbance.
- Weight gain.
- Sedation.
- Thyroid enlargement, hypothyroidism.
- ECG changes.
- Benign leukocytosis.
- Lithium is associated with an increased risk of **Ebstein's anomaly**, a cardiac defect in babies born to mothers taking lithium, although the absolute risk is very low. Weighed against the risk of untreated bipolar disorder, many women take lithium during pregnancy.

Anticonvulsants

CARBAMAZEPINE (TEGRETOL)

- Especially useful in treating mania with *mixed features* and *rapid-cycling* bipolar disorder; less effective for the depressed phase.
- Acts by blocking sodium channels and inhibiting action potentials.
- Onset of action is 5–7 days.
- Must check pregnancy test prior to initiating therapy as it increases the risk of neural tube defects.
- Carries risk of rash, SIADH, hyponatremia, benign leukopenia, and aplastic anemia (rare).
- CBC, LFTs must be obtained before initiating treatment and regularly monitored during treatment.
- Carbamazepine induces its own metabolism. Patients may therefore need a dose increase in the first few weeks to months.
  - Serum carbamazepine levels should be measured initially and after every few weeks for the first several months. Therapeutic level is 8–12 mcg/mL.

Side Effects
- The most common side effects are GI and CNS (e.g., drowsiness, ataxia, sedation, confusion).
- Potential dangerous skin rash (**Stevens–Johnson syndrome**).
- Leukopenia, hyponatremia, aplastic anemia, thrombocytopenia, and agranulocytosis.
- Elevation of liver enzymes, causing hepatitis.
- **Teratogenic** effects when used during pregnancy (neural tube defects).
- Significant drug interactions with many medications metabolized by the cytochrome P450 pathway, including inducing its own metabolism through *autoinduction* (requiring increasing dosages).
- Toxicity: Confusion, stupor, motor restlessness, ataxia, tremor, nystagmus, twitching, and vomiting.

KEY FACT

When prescribing lithium, it is important to monitor lithium levels, creatinine, and thyroid function tests. To remember labs for lithium:
P THY BEER
Pregnancy
Thyroid
Benign leukocytosis
Electrolytes
EKG
Renal

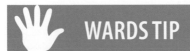

WARDS TIP

Blood levels are useful for lithium, valproic acid, carbamazepine, and clozapine. Remember the 8–12 rule for therapeutic windows of lithium (0.8–1.2), carbamazepine (8–12), and valproic acid (80–120).

WARDS TIP

The following factors increase Li+ levels:
- NSAIDs (e.g., ibuprofen)
- Aspirin (+/–)
- Thiazide diuretics
- Dehydration
- Salt deprivation
- Sweating (salt loss)
- Impaired renal function

KEY FACT

Carbamazepine is like "PacMan": It causes the CYP450 enzyme to chew up medications, resulting in low medication levels and requiring higher dosages than usual.

WARDS TIP

Lithium's side effect of leukocytosis can be advantageous when combined with other medications that decrease WBC count (e.g., clozapine).

WARDS QUESTION

Q: What is a potential consequence of using benzodiazepines (BDZ) with alcohol?
A: BDZs can be lethal when mixed with alcohol. Respiratory depression may cause death.

WARDS TIP

In chronic alcoholics or those with liver disease, use benzodiazepines that are not metabolized by the liver. There are a **LOT** of them:
Lorazepam
Oxazepam
Temazepam

VALPROIC ACID (DEPAKOTE AND DEPAKENE)

- Useful in treating acute mania, mania with mixed features, and rapid cycling.
- Multiple mechanisms of action: Blocks sodium channels and increases GABA concentrations in the brain.
- Comes in PO (Depakote), liquid (Depakene), and IV formulations.
- Monitoring of LFTs and CBC is necessary.
- Drug levels should be checked after 4–5 days. Therapeutic range is 80–120 µg/mL.
- Contraindicated in pregnancy, so care should be given in women of childbearing age (neural tube defects).
- Side effects include GI distress, sedation, cognitive slowing, weight gain, LFT elevations, hyperammonemia, thrombocytopenia, pancreatitis.

Lamotrigine (Lamictal)

- Efficacy for **bipolar depression**, though little efficacy for acute mania or prevention of mania.
- Believed to work on sodium channels that modulate glutamate and aspartate.
- Most common side effects are dizziness, sedation, headaches, and ataxia.
- Most serious side effect is **Stevens–Johnson syndrome** (life-threatening rash involving skin and mucous membranes) in 0.1%. This is most likely in the first 2–8 weeks, but is minimized by starting with *low* doses and increasing *slowly*.
- Valproate will increase lamotrigine levels, and lamotrigine will decrease valproate levels.

Oxcarbazepine (Trileptal)

- As effective in mood disorders as carbamazepine, but better tolerated.
- Less risk of rash and hepatic toxicity.
- Monitor sodium levels for hyponatremia.

Gabapentin (Neurontin)

- Often used adjunctively to help with anxiety, sleep, neuropathic pain.
- Little efficacy in bipolar disorder.

Pregabalin (Lyrica)

- Used in GAD (second-line) and fibromyalgia.
- Little efficacy in bipolar disorder.

Tiagabine (Gabitril): Questionable benefit in treating anxiety
Topiramate (Topamax)

- May be helpful with impulse control disorders.
- Beneficial side effect is **weight loss**.
- Can cause hypochloremic, metabolic acidosis as well as kidney stones.
- The most limiting side effect is **cognitive slowing** and sleepiness resulting in its nickname, "Dope-a-max."

Anxiolytics/Hypnotics

- Include benzodiazepines (BDZs), barbiturates, and buspirone.
- Common indications for anxiolytics/hypnotics include:
  - Anxiety disorders.
  - Muscle spasm.
  - Seizures.
  - Sleep disorders.
  - Alcohol withdrawal.
  - Anesthesia induction.

BENZODIAZEPINES

- BDZs are the most widely prescribed psychotropic medications.
- BDZs work by potentiating the effects of gamma-aminobutyric acid (GABA).
- They reduce anxiety and can be used to treat akathisia.
- Many patients become physically dependent on these medications and require increasing amounts for the same clinical effect (i.e., tolerance).
- Potential for abuse.
- Choice of BDZ is based on time to onset of action, duration of action, and method of metabolism.
- Relatively safer in overdose than barbiturates.
- **Long acting (half-life: >20 hours)**
  - **Diazepam (Valium):**
    - Rapid onset.
    - Used during detoxification from alcohol or sedative-hypnotic-anxiolytics, and for seizures.
    - Effective for muscle spasm.
    - Less commonly prescribed to treat anxiety because of euphoria.
  - **Clonazepam (Klonopin):**
    - Treatment of anxiety, including panic attacks.
    - Avoid with renal dysfunction; longer half-life allows for once or twice daily dosing.
- **Intermediate acting (half-life: 6–20 hours)**
  - **Alprazolam (Xanax):**
    - Treatment of anxiety, including panic attacks.
    - Short onset of action leads to euphoria, high abuse potential.
  - **Lorazepam (Ativan):**
    - Treatment of panic attacks, alcohol and sedative-hypnotic-anxiolytic detoxification, agitation.
    - Not metabolized by liver.
    - Used with haloperidol in IM formulations to quickly sedate agitated patients.
  - **Oxazepam (Serax):**
    - Alcohol and sedative-hypnotic-anxiolytic detoxification.
    - Not metabolized by liver.

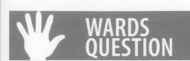

WARDS QUESTION

Q: How is benzodiazepine (BDZ) overdose treated?

A: Flumazenil; however, be careful not to induce withdrawal too quickly—this can be life threatening.

- **Temazepam (Restoril):**
  - Because of dependence, rarely used for treatment of insomnia.
  - Not metabolized by liver.
- **Short acting (half-life: <6 hours)**
  - **Midazolam (Versed):**
    - **Very short half-life**.
    - Primarily used in medical and surgical settings.

Side Effects

- Drowsiness.
- Impairment of intellectual function.
- Reduced motor coordination (careful in elderly).
- Anterograde amnesia.
- Withdrawal can be life threatening and cause seizures.
- Toxicity: Respiratory depression in overdose, especially when combined with alcohol.

NON-BDZ HYPNOTICS

- **Zolpidem (Ambien)/Zaleplon (Sonata)/Eszopiclone (Lunesta):**
  - Work by selective receptor binding to the omega-1 receptor on the GABA-A receptor, which is responsible for sedation.
  - Should be used for short-term treatment of insomnia.
  - Compared to BDZs, less tolerance/dependence occurs with prolonged use (but still can occur).
  - Zaleplon has a shorter half-life than zolpidem, which has a shorter half-life than eszopiclone.
  - Reports of anterograde amnesia, hallucinations, parasomnias (e.g., sleepwalking, sleepeating), increased fall risk, and GI side effects may limit their tolerability.
- **Diphenhydramine (Benadryl):**
  - An antihistamine with moderate anticholinergic effects.
  - Side effects include sedation, dry mouth, constipation, urinary retention, and blurry vision.
- **Ramelteon (Rozerem):**
  - Selective melatonin MT_1 and MT_2 agonist.
  - No tolerance or dependence, making it an effective and safe sleep aid.

NON-BDZ ANXIOLYTICS

- **Buspirone (BuSpar):**
  - Partial agonist at 5HT-1A receptor, thereby decreasing serotonergic activity.
  - Slower onset of action than BDZs (takes several weeks for effect).
  - Not considered as effective as other options, and so it is often used in combination with another agent (e.g., an SSRI) for the treatment of generalized anxiety disorder.
  - Does not potentiate the CNS depression of alcohol (useful in alcoholics), and has a low potential for abuse/addiction.
  - Dosed three times per day.

- **Hydroxyzine (Atarax):**
  - An antihistamine.
  - Side effects include sedation, dry mouth, constipation, urinary retention, and blurry vision.
  - Useful for patients who want quick-acting, short-term medication, but who cannot take BDZs for various reasons.
- **Barbiturates** (e.g., **butalbitol, phenobarbital, amobarbitol, pentobarbital**): Rarely used because of the lethality of overdose, significant withdrawal, potential for abuse, and side-effect profile.
- **Propranolol:**
  - Beta-blocker.
  - Useful in treating the autonomic effects of panic attacks or social phobia (i.e., performance anxiety), such as palpitations, sweating, and tachycardia.
  - Also used to treat akathisia (side effect of antipsychotics).

Psychostimulants

Used in ADHD and in treatment refractory depression.

- **Dextroamphetamine and amphetamines (Dexedrine, Adderall):**
  - Dextroamphetamine is the D-isomer of amphetamine.
  - Schedule II due to high potential for **abuse/diversion**.
  - Monitor BP, and watch for weight loss, insomnia, exacerbation of tics, decreased seizure threshold.
- **Methylphenidate (Ritalin, Concerta):**
  - CNS stimulant, similar to amphetamine.
  - Schedule II.
  - Watch for leukopenia or anemia.
  - Monitor BP and CBC with differential, and watch for weight loss, insomnia, exacerbation of tics, decreased seizure threshold.
- **Atomoxetine (Strattera):**
  - Inhibits presynaptic norepinephrine reuptake, resulting in increased synaptic norepinephrine and dopamine.
  - Less appetite suppression and insomnia.
  - Not classified as a controlled substance.
  - Less abuse potential than dextroamphetamine/methylphenidate but less effective.
  - Rare liver toxicity, and possible increase in suicidal ideation in children/adolescents.
- **Modafinil (Provigil):** Used in narcolepsy, not ADHD.

Cognitive Enhancers

Used in major neurocognitive disorders (dementias).

ACETYLCHOLINESTERASE INHIBITORS

- **Donepezil (Aricept):**
  - Once-daily dosing.
  - Some GI side effects.
  - Used in mild-to-moderate neurocognitive disorders (dementias).

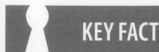

KEY FACT

Alzheimer medications, such as donepezil and rivastigmine, work by reversible inhibition of acetylcholine esterase.

- **Galantamine (Razadyne):**
  - Twice-daily dosing.
  - GI side effects.
  - Used in mild-to-moderate neurocognitive disorders (dementias).
- **Rivastigmine (Exelon):**
  - Twice-daily dosing.
  - Has daily patch form, with fewer side effects.
  - Used in mild-to-moderate neurocognitive disorders (dementias).

NMDA (GLUTAMATE) RECEPTOR ANTAGONIST

- **Memantine (Namenda):**
  - Used in moderate-to-severe neurocognitive disorders (dementia).
  - Fewer side effects than cholinesterase inhibitors.
  - Should be used in conjunction with acetylcholinesterase inhibitor.

Reference List of Medications That May Cause Psychiatric Symptoms

PSYCHOSIS

Sympathomimetics, analgesics, antibiotics (e.g., isoniazid, antimalarials), anticholinergics, anticonvulsants, antihistamines, corticosteroids, antiparkinsonian agents.

AGITATION/CONFUSION/DELIRIUM

Antipsychotics, **anticholinergics**, **antihistamines**, antidepressants, antiarrhythmics, antineoplastics, corticosteroids, NSAIDs, antiasthmatics, antibiotics, antihypertensives, antiparkinsonian agents, thyroid hormones.

DEPRESSION

Antihypertensives, antiparkinsonian agents, **corticosteroids**, calcium channel blockers, NSAIDs, antibiotics, peptic ulcer drugs.

ANXIETY

Sympathomimetics, antiasthmatics, antiparkinsonian agents, hypoglycemic agents, NSAIDs, thyroid hormones.

SEDATION/POOR CONCENTRATION

Antianxiety agents/hypnotics, anticholinergics, mood stabilizers, antibiotics, antihistamines, antipsychotics (e.g., clozapine, quetiapine, olanzapine).

SELECTED MEDICATIONS

- **Procainamide, quinidine:** Confusion, delirium.
- **Albuterol:** Anxiety, confusion.
- **Isoniazid:** Psychosis.

- **Tetracycline:** Depression.
- **Nifedipine, verapamil:** Depression.
- **Cimetidine:** Depression, confusion, psychosis.
- **Steroids:** Aggressiveness/agitation, mania, depression, anxiety, psychosis.

Other Treatments

ELECTROCONVULSIVE THERAPY (ECT)

Patients are often premedicated with atropine, and then given general anesthesia and muscle relaxants (e.g., succinylcholine). A generalized tonic-clonic seizure is then induced using unilateral or bilateral electrodes placed on the head. While the mechanism of action of ECT is not fully known, there are likely anticonvulsant effects, as well as brain perfusion and connectivity changes involved. ECT is **the most effective** treatment for major depressive disorder, especially with psychotic features, as well as for acute mania and catatonia. It is often used in patients who cannot tolerate medications or who have failed other treatments. ECT is discontinued after symptomatic improvement, typically a course of 8–12 sessions given three times weekly. Monthly *maintenance ECT* is often used to prevent relapse of symptoms, and the addition of nortriptyline or venlafaxine may prolong remission even further. The most common side effects are muscle soreness, headaches, amnesia, and confusion. Bilateral electrode placement is more efficacious, but increases memory impairment and confusion. Evidence shows that the memory loss is almost always temporary and returns to baseline at 6 months.

DEEP BRAIN STIMULATION (DBS)

DBS is a surgical treatment involving the implantation of a medical device that sends electrical impulses to specific parts of the brain. DBS in select brain regions has provided benefits for Parkinson disease and disabling dystonia, as well as for chronic pain and tremors. Its underlying principles and mechanisms are still not clear. DBS directly changes brain activity in a controlled manner and its effects are reversible (unlike those of lesioning techniques). DBS has been used to treat various affective disorders, including major depression. While DBS has proven helpful for some patients, there is potential for serious complications and side effects.

REPETITIVE TRANSCRANIAL MAGNETIC STIMULATION (rTMS)

rTMS is a noninvasive method to excite neurons in the brain. Weak electric currents are induced in the tissue by rapidly changing magnetic fields, a process called electromagnetic induction. In this way, brain activity can be triggered with minimal discomfort. rTMS can produce longer-lasting changes than nonrepetitive stimulation. Numerous small-scale studies have demonstrated efficacy in the treatment of major depression; however, studies show less efficacy than for ECT, and the price of treatment is high. Side effects include seizures (rare), as well as headache and scalp pain.

LIGHT THERAPY

Light therapy, or phototherapy, consists of exposure to daylight or to specific wavelengths of light using lasers, light-emitting diodes, fluorescent lamps, dichroic lamps or very bright, full-spectrum light, for a prescribed amount of time and, in some cases, at a specific time of day. The recommendation is for using a 10,000 lux bright white light for 30 minutes per day in the early morning. Light therapy is used to treat major depression with a seasonal pattern (**seasonal affective disorder**), with some support for its use with nonseasonal psychiatric disorders.

KETAMINE INFUSION

Ketamine is an NMDA receptor antagonist that is most commonly used as an anesthetic agent. Ketamine can be given as an IV infusion for the treatment of unipolar major depression. It's effect is rapid (with response within 40–120 minutes), but the effect dissipates by day 10–14. Ketamine carries a risk of dissociation/psychosis, bladder toxicity, and neurotoxicity. Currently, use of IV ketamine for depression is still mostly limited to research settings, but increasingly through specialized ketamine clinics. Esketamine, the intranasal formulation of ketamine, was recently FDA approved for treatment-resistant depression.

Most Common Psychiatric Medications for Wards

Typical Antipsychotics (D2 antagonism)

Drug name (Brand)	Dosing	Side Effects	Monitoring	Other
chlorpromazine (Thorazine)	200–800 mg	Hypotension, sedation, orthostasis	EKG, BMI, QTc	Least potent PO, IM
fluphenazine (Prolixin)	6–20 mg	EPS, sedation		PO, IM, LAI
haloperidol (Haldol)	2–20 mg	EPS, sedation		PO, IM, LAI
perphenazine (Triaflon)	8–32 mg	EPS, sedation		PO, IM

Watch for NMS (fever, **lead pipe rigidity**).

EPS tx: **Akathisia** (propranolol 10 mg TID), **Parkinsonism/Dystonia** (benztropine 1–2 mg daily)

Atypical Antipsychotics (D2 and 5HT2a antagonism)

Drug name (Brand)	Dosing	Side Effects	Monitoring	Other
clozapine (Clozaril)	300–900 mg	Anticholinergic, orthostatis, agranulocytosis, drooling	Weekly ANC	Most efficacious Lower suicide risk
aripiprazole (Abilify)	5–30 mg	Akathisia	**For all: A1C, fasting glucose, lipid profile, BMI, LFTs, renal function**	PO and LAI
lurasidone (Latuda)	40–120 mg	Akathisia		Give with food
olanzapine (Zyprexa)	10–30 mg	Metabolic syndrome, orthostasis, sedating		PO, IM, LAI
paliperidone (Invega)	3–12 mg	Hyperprolactinemia, EPS, sedation, metabolic syndrome		PO and LAI
quetiapine (Seroquel)	50–800 mg	Metabolic syndrome, orthostasis, sedating		PO, check QTc
risperidone (Risperdal)	2–6 mg	Hyperprolactinemia, EPS, sedation, metabolic syndrome		PO and LAI

Mood Stabilizers

Drug name Brand)	Dosing	Side Effects	Monitoring	Other
Lithium	900–1800 mg	GI upset, tremor, nephrogenic DI, renal failure	Thyroid, renal, serum drug level (0.8–1.2)	Ebstein's anomaly Lower suicide risk
lamotrigine (Lamictal)	100–200 mg	GI upset, SJS rash	Monitor for rash	Dose slowly
valproic acid (Depakote)	500–2000 mg	GI upset, weight gain, liver toxicity	Liver, ammonia, serum drug level (80–120)	Contraindicated in pregnancy: neural tube defect
carbamazepine (Tegretol)	800–1600 mg	Hyponatremia, agranulocytosis	Liver, renal, serum drug level (8–10)	Contraindicated in pregnancy: neural tube defect PacMan inducer

Antidepressants

Drug name (Brand)	Dosing	Side Effects/Monitor	Other
fluoxetine (Prozac)	20–80 mg	SSRI's: GI upset, sexual dysfunction, bleeding, discontinuation syndrome	Long half-life
sertraline (Zoloft)	50–200 mg		Safe in pregnancy
escitalopram (Lexapro)	10–20 mg		Few med interactions
venlafaxine (Effexor)	75–225 mg	Tremor, HTN, akathisia	Short half-life
duloxetine (Cymbalta)	40–120 mg	Monitor LFTs	Treats pain, fibromyalgia
mirtazapine (Remeron)	15–45 mg	Sedation, weight gain	Activating at higher doses
buproprion (Wellbutrin)	150–450 mg	Activating, insomnia	Increased seizure risk

Watch for 5HT syndrome (Fever, **hyperreflexia**, **myoclonus**, GI disturbance)

NOTES

CHAPTER 19

FORENSIC PSYCHIATRY

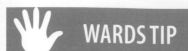

WARDS TIP

A wrong prediction or a bad outcome is not necessarily proof of malpractice.

KEY FACT

Four **D**s of malpractice: **D**ereliction of **D**uty that was the **D**irect cause of **D**amage.

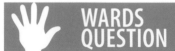

WARDS QUESTION

Q: What legal case set the precedent that physicians have a duty to report patients who are potentially dangerous to others?
A: *Tarasoff v. Regents of the University of California* which called for the *duty to warn.*

KEY FACT

Doctors are required to report child abuse, but lawyers are not.

Forensic psychiatry is a medical subspecialty that includes areas in which psychiatry is applied to legal matters. Forensic psychiatrists often conduct evaluations requested by the court or attorneys.

While some forensic psychiatrists specialize exclusively in legal issues, almost all psychiatrists have to work within one of the many spheres where the mental health and legal system overlap. These areas include the following:

- Risk assessment.
- Criminal responsibility.
- Competence/Decisional capacity.
- Child custody and visitation.
- Trauma.
- Mental disability.
- Malpractice.
- Involuntary treatment.
- Correctional psychiatry.

Legal issues are considered **criminal** in nature if someone is being charged with a crime. **Civil** cases involve other kinds of rights and may result in monetary awards. It is important to note that the specific laws pertaining to the various topics discussed in this chapter may vary by state.

Standard of Care and Malpractice

- The **standard of care** in psychiatry is generally defined as the skill level and knowledge base of the average, prudent psychiatrist in a given community.
- **Negligence** is practicing below the standard of care.
- **Malpractice** is the act of being negligent as a doctor.
- The following four conditions typically must be proven by a preponderance of the evidence in order to sustain a claim of malpractice:
  1. The physician had a duty of care (psychiatrist–patient relationship).
  2. The physician breached their duty by practice that did not meet the standard of care (negligence).
  3. The patient was harmed.
  4. The harm was directly caused by the physician's negligence.
- If a malpractice case is successful, the patient can receive **compensatory damages** (reimbursement for medical expenses, lost salary, or physical suffering) and **punitive damages** (money awarded to "punish" the doctor).

Confidentiality

All information regarding a doctor–patient relationship should be held confidential, except when otherwise exempted by statute, such as:

- When sharing relevant information with other staff members who are also treating the patient.
- If subpoenaed—Physician must supply all requested information.
- If child abuse is suspected—Obligated to report to the proper authorities.
- If a patient is suicidal—Physician may need to admit the patient, with or without the patient's consent, and share information with the hospital staff.
- If a patient threatens direct harm to another person—Physician may have a duty to warn the intended victim.

Decision Making

- Process by which patients knowingly and voluntarily agree to a treatment or procedure.
- In order to make informed decisions, patients must know the purpose of the treatment, alternative treatments, and the potential risks and benefits of undergoing and of refusing the treatment.
- The patient should have the opportunity to ask questions.
- Situations that do not require informed consent:
  - Lifesaving medical emergency.
  - Prevention of suicidal or homicidal behavior.
  - Unemancipated minors (typically require informed consent from the parent or legal guardian).

EMANCIPATED MINORS

- Considered competent to give consent for all medical care without parental input or consent.
- Minors are considered emancipated if they are:
  - Self-supporting.
  - In the military.
  - Married.
  - Have children **or pregnant.**

 A 74-year-old male with insulin-dependent diabetes mellitus and severe major depressive disorder was admitted to the intensive care unit for treatment of diabetic ketoacidosis. The internal medicine team calls your psychiatry consult-liaison service to evaluate the patient for depression and provide treatment recommendations.

When you meet the patient, he is disoriented, confused, and has a waxing and waning level of consciousness. His mini-mental state exam (MMSE) score is 18/30. You identify that the patient is likely delirious, and you are unable to obtain any useful historical information. After interviewing the patient's daughter by phone, you learn that the patient's wife passed away 2 years ago, and in the past he had told family members that he can no longer live without her. One year ago, his daughter found him in the garage taping a hose to his car's exhaust pipe. She said that he broke down crying and admitted that he was going to kill himself by carbon monoxide poisoning. His daughter has been very concerned because he refuses to check his glucose or take his insulin as recommended. She stated, "I think he was trying to kill himself by not taking care of his diabetes."

He is followed daily by your consult-liaison team, and his MMSE score improves to 28/30. On hospital day 5, the internal medicine team informs you that he has developed wet gangrene in his right lower extremity and will need to have a below-knee amputation as soon as possible. The team asks you to assess the patient's capacity to make medical decisions because he is adamantly refusing to consent to this procedure.

You meet with the patient to discuss his medical situation. He is alert, lucid, and fully oriented. His affect is euthymic and appropriate. He states, "My doctor told me that I had an ulcer on my foot from poorly controlled diabetes that has become severely infected. I was told that I need to have my right

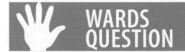

WARDS QUESTION

Q: In what situations is informed consent not required?
A: In a lifesaving medical emergency, to prevent suicide or homicide, or when treating an unemancipated minor.

KEY FACT

Elements of informed consent (4 Rs):

- **R**eason for treatment
- **R**isks and benefits
- **R**easonable alternatives
- **R**efused treatment consequences

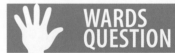

WARDS QUESTION

Q: What is the key difference between capacity and competency?
A: Capacity is a clinical term assessed by physicians, while competency is a legal term decided by a judge.

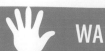

WARDS TIP

When evaluating for decision-making capacity think **CURA**:
Communicate a clear choice
Understand the situation, proposed treatment, and treatment alternatives
Reason logically through information and decision
Appreciate consequences, including risk/benefits of treatment or refusal of treatment

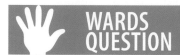

WARDS QUESTION

Q: What is the standard hierarchy for choosing a surrogate decision maker?
A: 1. Durable POA or court-appointed guardian
2. Spouse
3. Adult offspring
4. Parent
5. Sibling
6. Other relative in close contact with patient
7. Close friend

KEY FACT

Emancipated minors do not need parental consent to make medical decisions.

leg amputated very soon or else I could die from the infection." He maintains that he is not interested in the surgical procedure that has been recommended. He adds, "My daughter is begging me to have the surgery, but I'm already old and I don't want to have to use a prosthetic leg or a wheelchair. I do not think life would be worth living if I had this amputation." He denies suicidal thoughts, plan, or intent.

Does this patient with history of severe major depressive disorder demonstrate the capacity to refuse a potentially lifesaving procedure?

Yes, he demonstrates the capacity to refuse the recommended amputation. Legal standards for decision-making capacity to consent or refuse medical treatment involve the following: the ability to communicate a choice, to understand the relevant information, to appreciate the medical consequences of the situation, and to reason about treatment choices. In this case, the patient demonstrated the ability to discuss all of these topics. Although he was cognitively impaired on admission, his delirium eventually cleared.

However, the case is complicated by the fact that the patient may be currently suffering from major depression. This should be further assessed. While a history of current major depression does not preclude having decisional capacity, the patient should be evaluated carefully to ensure that his refusal of treatment does not stem from intent to commit suicide. If it does, then his suicidal intent would be interfering with his ability to reason. Optimally, the consult-liaison team may recommend treating the depression and readdressing the surgical procedure when his depression is in remission, but this may take many weeks and failure to amputate the limb in a timely manner could result in death. Since the patient demonstrates decision-making capacity and does not appear to be suicidal at this time, the medical team must respect the patient's wishes and treat the condition without surgery

DECISIONAL CAPACITY

Competence and *capacity* are terms that refer to a patient's ability to make informed treatment decisions.

- *Capacity* is a clinical term and may be assessed by physicians.
- *Competence* is a legal term and can be decided only by a judge.
- Decisional capacity is *task specific* and can fluctuate over time.
- In order for a patient to have decisional capacity, they must be able to:
  - Understand the relevant information regarding treatment (purpose, risks, benefits).
  - Appreciate the appropriate weight and impact of the decision.
  - Logically manipulate the information to make a decision.
  - Communicate a choice or preference.
  - Criteria for determining capacity may be more stringent if the consequences of a patient's decision are very serious.
- If a patient is determined not to have decisional capacity, the decision is typically made by a surrogate decision maker, usually a power of attorney, spouse, or close family member.

GUARDIANS AND CONSERVATORS

- May be appointed by a judge to make treatment decisions for incompetent patients.

- Make decisions by "substituted judgment." This means making decisions based on what the patient would most likely have wanted, were the patient competent.
- Patients can express their wishes for treatment in advance of losing competence or capacity using a mental health advance directive form called "Declaration for Mental Health Treatment."

Admission to a Psychiatric Hospital

The two main categories of admission to a psychiatric hospital are voluntary and involuntary.

- **Voluntary:**
  - Patient requests or agrees to be admitted to the psychiatric ward.
  - Voluntary patients often have to meet the same symptom severity criteria as involuntary patients as listed below.
  - Voluntary patients may not have the right to be discharged *immediately* upon request.
  - Patient must have capacity and be competent to be admitted as a voluntary patient to an inpatient facility.
- **Involuntary:**
  - Patient must be found to be imminently at risk of harm to one's self or others or unable to provide for their basic needs.
  - Involuntary patients have legal rights to a trial to challenge their hospitalization.
  - Involuntary patients do not automatically lose the right to refuse treatment, including the involuntary administration of nonemergent medication.
  - Involuntary commitment is supported by legal principles of **police power** (protecting citizens from each other) and **parens patriae** (protecting citizens who can't care for themselves).

Disability

- **Mental impairment:** Any mental or psychological disorder.
- **Mental disability:** Alteration of an individual's capacity to meet personal, social, or occupational demands due to a mental impairment.
- To assess whether an impairment is also a disability, consider four categories:
  - Activities of daily living.
  - Social functioning.
  - Concentration, persistence, and pace.
  - Deterioration or decompensation in work settings.

Competence to Stand Trial

- *Competence* is a legal term for the capacity to understand, rationally manipulate, and apply information to make a reasoned decision on a specific issue. This definition varies by state.

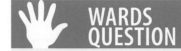

WARDS QUESTION

Q: When can a patient be involuntarily hospitalized on a psychiatric unit?
A: When they pose a risk of harm to self, others, or cannot provide for their basic needs.

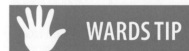

WARDS TIP

If a child presents to the emergency department with various bruises, suspicious injuries in various stages of healing, and numerous prior emergency room visits, your next step would most likely be to contact the appropriate authorities.

KEY FACT

Sixth Amendment: Right to counsel, a speedy trial, and to confront witnesses.

KEY FACT

Fourteenth Amendment: Right to due process of law.

The fact that someone is mentally ill doesn't mean they aren't competent to stand trial.

- The Sixth and Fourteenth Amendments to the Constitution are the basis for the law that someone cannot be tried if they are not mentally competent to stand trial.
- This was established by the legal case *Dusky v. United States* in 1960.
- If a defendant has significant mental health problems or behaves irrationally in court, their competency to stand trial should be considered.
- Competence to stand trial may change over time.
- To stand trial, a defendant must:
  - Understand the charges against them.
  - Be familiar with the courtroom personnel and procedure.
  - Have the ability to work with an attorney and participate in their trial.
  - Understand possible consequences.

Not Guilty by Reason of Insanity (NGRI)

- Conviction of a crime requires both an "evil deed" (*actus reus*) and "evil intent" (*mens rea*).
- **Insanity** is a legal term, and its definition varies by state (see Table 19-1).
- If someone is declared legally insane, they are not criminally responsible for their act.
- Some states have a ruling of Guilty but Mentally Ill (GBMI) instead of NGRI, or no criminal insanity defense at all.
- NGRI is used in less than 1% of criminal cases.
- It is successful in 26% of cases that continue to use it throughout the trial.
- Those found NGRI often spend the same amount of time (or more) as involuntary psychiatric patients than they would have spent in prison if they were found guilty.

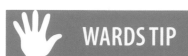

After John Hinckley received NGRI for an assassination attempt on President Reagan, there was public outcry against lenient NGRI standards, contributing to the Insanity Defense Reform Act of 1984.

Risk Assessment

- Mental disorders are neither necessary nor sufficient causes of violence.
- The major risk factors of violence are a history of violence, being young, male, and of lower socioeconomic status.
- Substance use is a major determinant of violence, whether it occurs in the context of a mental illness or not.

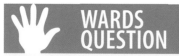

Q: What is the most important factor in assessing a patient's risk of violence?
A: The individual's history of violence.

TABLE 19-1. Insanity Defense Standards	
Standard	**Definition**
M'Naghten	■ Person did not understand what they were doing *or* its wrongfulness. ■ Most stringent test.
American Law Institute (ALI) Model Penal Code	Person could neither appreciate the criminality of their conduct *nor* conform their conduct to the requirements of the law.
Irresistible Impulse	Person could not appreciate right from wrong *or* could not control actions.
Durham	■ The person's criminal act has resulted from mental illness. ■ Most lenient test and is rarely used.

- **Predicting dangerousness:**
  - Short term easier than long term.
  - High false positives because of low base rates (most people are not violent).

Malingering

- Feigning or exaggerating symptoms for "secondary gain," including:
  - Financial gain (injury law suit).
  - Avoiding school, work, or other responsibilities.
  - Obtaining medications of abuse (opioids, benzodiazepines).
  - Avoiding legal consequences.
- Signs for detecting malingering:
  - Atypical presentation.
  - "Textbook" description of the illness.
  - History of working in the medical field.
  - Symptoms that are present only when the patient knows they are being observed.
  - History of substance use or antisocial personality disorder.
  - Reluctant to engage in invasive/in-depth testing or treatment.

Child and Family Law

Evaluations for which a child forensic psychiatrist may be needed include:

- Child custody.
- Termination of parental rights.
- Child abuse or neglect.

Correctional Psychiatry

- With the closing of state psychiatric hospitals (i.e., deinstitutionalization), many persons with mental illness have moved to correctional institutions.
- Psychiatrists who practice in jails and prisons must balance treating the inmates as their patients and maintaining safety in the institution.
- Issues of **confidentiality** and **violence** are key.

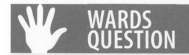

WARDS QUESTION

Q: What is the key difference between malingering and factitious disorder?
A: The motivation for malingering is for *secondary gain* (external motivations, such as avoiding work or jail), whereas factitious disorder is *primary gain* (internal motivations, such as to assume the sick-role).

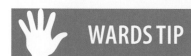

WARDS TIP

The contribution of people with mental illness to overall rates of violence is small. Those with mental illness are more likely to be the *victims* of violence than the perpetrators.

NOTES

CHAPTER 20

APPROACH TO THE PSYCHIATRIC PATIENT IN THE
EMERGENCY DEPARTMENT

Safety Assessment

During the course of your psychiatry clerkship, you may be asked to see a patient who is in the Emergency Department (ED). Unlike on the psychiatry floor/ward or even a psychiatric emergency holding unit, the ED sees patients with all sorts of complaints, and is not particularly well-suited for psychiatric patients. Reasons contributing to the ED environment being challenging include staff frequently entering and exiting the patient's room, which may interrupt your interview; a high level of activity and noise; and a large number of distractions. Psychiatric patients in the ED are from some of the most marginalized segments of society. They may be homeless, may have untreated, undertreated or mistreated psychiatric illness, and their presentation may be confounded by acute intoxication with alcohol, drugs, or co-existing medical illness.

Many patients are brought in by law enforcement/police, which may unfortunately exacerbate a patient's aggression or paranoia. When patients are hostile or scared, it is difficult to develop a rapport with them.

When interviewing such patients, it is preferable to enter the room without law enforcement as long as there does not seem to be an immediate threat of physical harm to you or your team (see Figure 20-1).

How to assess whether the room/patient is safe (see Table 20-1):

- Position yourself on the patient's nondominant side
  - This is usually the patient's left in 95% of cases.
  - Patients usually wear their watch on their nondominant hand.
  - Their belt buckle usually faces to the nondominant side.
- Position yourself close to the exit
- Do a quick visual to make sure no objects that can be used as weapons are around. ED rooms designated as psychiatric rooms are usually devoid of such objects, but if the patient is in a regular medical room, then there may be many items that could be dangerous (e.g., suction canisters, trashcans, needles, intravenous [IV] poles).

Medical Clearance Orders

- De-escalating the situation:
- Be prepared to de-escalate the situation. Recognize that the patient may not be there by choice; that they may be been treated poorly by law enforcement; that they fear losing their independence; that this new environment aggravates their paranoia; and that the ED may be a place that they mistrust.

De-escalation Techniques

- Speak softly (if they have to strain to hear you, they will have to be quiet themselves).
- Offer them food or drink (they rarely have to go to surgery, so keeping them NPO is not usually a concern, and most ED psychiatric patients are hungry).
- Bring them a blanket (it is usually cold in the ED).

FIGURE 20-1. Suggested steps for approaching a psychiatric patient in the ED.

TABLE 20-1. Typical Medical "Clearance" Orders
Undress patient, place in hospital gown
Continuous pulse oximetry
Cardiac monitor
Electrocardiogram (ECG)
Peripheral IV
Complete blood count (CBC)
Complete metabolic panel (electrolytes and liver function tests)
b-hCG (if female)
Magnesium
Alcohol
Salicylate
Acetaminophen
Urinalysis
Urine drug screen
Suicide precautions (sitter)
Seizure precautions (padded bedrails)

- *Speak to them like an individual.* Pick your favorite benign topic of conversation, such as the weather. One choice is: "Where were you born and raised?" It's unusual to be asked something like that, so it tends to catch the patient off guard and put them more into a conversation mode.

- *Ask their permission to examine them.* Respecting anyone's personal space is important, but especially so with the psychiatric patient.

- If they are going to be admitted to the psychiatric unit, *explain what is going to happen to them.* Hopefully they have been seen by an ED physician and the process has been discussed, but this is not always the case. If you are the first student they are talking to, explain that the ED will do a medical clearance evaluation (see Table 20-1), and then they will be brought to the behavioral health unit/psychiatry floor. While respecting their dignity and privacy, ED psychiatric patients should be placed in a gown and searched for items such as weapons, drugs, drug paraphernalia, and medication patches.

Communication with ED

Communicate with the ED team any plans you have made with your psychiatry attending.

- Let them know if there are any medications the patient should or should not receive.
- Expedite the patient's movement out of the ED if possible, as it is the least restful place for them.

Acutely Agitated Patients

In the event that an acutely agitated patient cannot be de-escalated, medication(s) may be required. The most common choice is an antipsychotic with or without a benzodiazepine. Either class can achieve control on its own, but benzodiazepines tend to be more sedating. Table 20-2 lists the most common medications used to control acute agitation in the ED. The ability to administer oral or intramuscular medications is very helpful as an acutely agitated patient may not cooperate for the team to safely place an IV.

Assessment of a Sleeping or Unresponsive Patient

If you walk in the room and the patient appears to be sleeping or unresponsive, you should do the following:

- Assess the patient's ABCs
  - Airway: Can the patient speak? (if yes, airway is patent)
  - Breathing: Is the patient breathing? (look for chest rise, auscultate lungs)
  - Circulation: Does the patient have a pulse? (auscultate heart, check blood pressure)
- If the patient's ABCs are compromised, immediately get an ED physician. Pull the panic cord if you need to.
- If the patient's ABCs are stable but they appear somnolent, explore with the ED team whether the patient has received any medications from the ED or paramedics/emergency medical services (EMS) which could be contributing.

Medication Interactions

Psychiatric medications can adversely interact with many other medications. Using a drug interaction calculator to verify interactions will be a huge service to your patient as well as your team. Do not assume that just because patient is prescribed a set of medications, that they are all safe to be taken together. Often, patients get prescriptions for various medications from several prescribers, and concurrent prescriptions are not cross-checked.

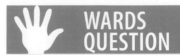

WARDS QUESTION

Q: What medication is used to reverse opiate/opioid overdose?
A: Naloxone.

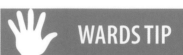

WARDS TIP

Case: You are called to the ED to see a patient. You encounter a 22-year-old male who is very agitated, trying to break free of the numerous paramedics and security officers trying to hold him down. He is loudly yelling to be let go as well as clearly responding to internal stimuli. How should you manage the situation?

Answer: Try verbally de-escalating the situation while you order chemical restraints. Order a benzodiazepine and an antipsychotic together, as that will result in less total benzodiazepine dose being needed.

KEY FACT

Flumazenil is used for benzodiazepine overdose reversal BUT its use can cause seizures, especially in those patients with a low seizure threshold. Use with caution, and have an airway cart ready in case airway control becomes necessary. Remember that benzodiazepine withdrawal can be life threatening.

TABLE 20-2. Common Medications Used in Adults for Control of Acute Agitation in the ED

Medication (Brand Name)	Drug Class	Initial Dose	Onset of Action (minutes)	Half-Life (hours)	Adverse Effects/Notes
Lorazepam (Ativan®)	Benzodiazepine	PO, IM, PR, IV: 2 mg	IM: 15 PO: 30–60	12	More sedating than antipsychotics alone
Midazolam (Versed®)	Benzodiazepine	PO, IM, IN, IV 2 mg	PO, IN: 12–15 IV: 2–5	1–3	Shortest onset of action Short duration of action may be both an advantage and disadvantage; intranasal route unique
Haloperidol	Typical (1st generation) antipsychotic	PO, IM, IV: 5 mg	15	20	Extrapyramidal symptoms; anticholinergic symptoms; QT prolongation; neuroleptic malignant syndrome
Olanzapine (Zyprexa®)	Atypical (2nd generation) antipsychotic	ODT: 5, 10, 15, 20 mg IM: 10 mg	15–60	20–50	Safety and efficacy not established for children less than 13 years. Life-threatening sedation and hypotension when co-administered with a benzodiazepine.
Ziprasidone (Geodon®)	Atypical (2nd generation) antipsychotic	IM; 20 mg	60	2–5	Causes QTc prolongation; important to assess known history of QTc prolongation, recent myocardial infarction, uncompensated heart failure, or if taking other medications known to prolong the QTc interval.
Risperidone (Risperdal®)	Atypical (2nd generation) antipsychotic	ODT and solution	IM: 30–60 PO: 60–120	20	
Quetiapine (Seroquel®)	Atypical (2nd generation) antipsychotic	Oral tablet form only	90	6	Long time of onset limits use in acute agitation

Causes of Mental Status Changes

Lab and vital sign abnormalities that can cause altered mental status or delirium:

- Hypoglycemia/Hyperglycemia.
- Hyponatremia/Hypernatremia.
- Hypocalcemia/Hypercalcemia.
- Hypothermia/Hyperthermia.
- Hypothyroidism.
- Hypovolemia.
- Hypercarbia.
- Hypoxemia.

KEY FACT

Geriatric patients (>65 years) are often sensitive to medications so it is recommended to start with smaller doses. Also some geriatric patients can have paradoxical agitation with benzodiazepines. Remember that it is unusual for a patient over age 40 to have a first episode of psychosis. Be sure to search for other medical causes of psychosis.

KEY FACT

Normal QTc—Men: <440 ms and women: <460 ms.
An increase in 10 ms is associated with a 5–7% increase in Torsades de pointes.

KEY FACT

Visual hallucinations should *always* prompt search for an underlying medical pathology. Although visual hallucinations can occur with psychiatric disorders, auditory hallucinations are more common.

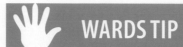

WARDS TIP

Case: You are called to the ED to see an elderly patient who you are told is psychotic. The patient has a history of Parkinson for which he takes carbidopa-levodopa. He had vomited earlier so he was given one oral dissolving tablet of ondansetron. The ED team wants to give him some Olanzapine to help control his symptoms. As the team that will take over the care of this patient, what would you advise?

Answer: Most anti-parkinsonian medications including carbidopa-levodopa can induce psychosis in Parkinson patients, usually manifested as visual hallucinations. It is the most common nonmotor disabling symptom in PD. A quick drug interaction search will reveal that carbidopa-levodopa has a serious interaction with olanzapine, in that it reduces the activity of carbidopa-levodopa. In addition, the combination of ondansetron and olanzapine can result in dangerously prolonged QTc, so be sure to check an ECG.

INDEX